SARS war

Combating the Disease

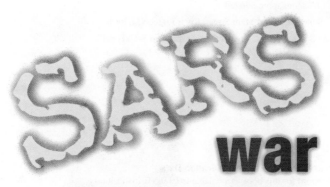

Editors

Leung Ping Chung
*Chinese University of Hong Kong and
Prince of Wales Hospital
Hong Kong*

Ooi Eng Eong
*The Environmental Health Institute,
National Environment Agency
Singapore*

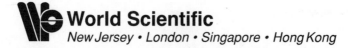

World Scientific
New Jersey • London • Singapore • Hong Kong

Published by

World Scientific Publishing Co. Pte. Ltd.

5 Toh Tuck Link, Singapore 596224

USA office: Suite 202, 1060 Main Street, River Edge, NJ 07661

UK office: 57 Shelton Street, Covent Garden, London WC2H 9HE

British Library Cataloguing-in-Publication Data
A catalogue record for this book is available from the British Library.

SARS WAR

ISBN 981-238-433-2
ISBN 981-238-438-3 (pbk)

Printed in Singapore.

CONTENTS

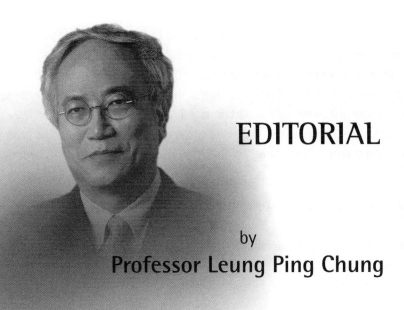

EDITORIAL

by
Professor Leung Ping Chung

Professor Leung Ping Chung, Hon DSocSc, DSc, FHKAM (Orthopaedics), FHKCOS, MS, FRACS, FRCS (Edin), MB BS, is a highly respected medical expert in Hong Kong. He is the Chairman of the Management Committee, Institute of Chinese Medicine, The Chinese University of Hong Kong. Professor Leung is one of the first doctors to propose using serum from recovered patients to treat SARS, and this method has so far produced optimistic results. His areas of expertise include orthopaedics, osteoporosis, surgery and traditional Chinese medicine.

SARS, which is now wreaking havoc in Asia, is a modern epidemic. Therefore, it is inappropriate to compare it with "The Plague" of the Middle Ages, because at that time the only cures available were in the form of witchcraft and herbal remedies. The plague outbreak subsequently led to a staggering death toll of 100 million. It is also inappropriate to compare it with the Ebola outbreak, another modern epidemic which only spread within the geographical limits of central Africa. Although this virus had claimed countless lives, it was swiftly contained. SARS could be more similar to the plague that occurred in the regions of Guangdong and Guangxi in China about a hundred years ago. Western medical science was already well established then, and cures were easily available. However, the fear engendered by

SARS does not seem to be less than that caused by the recorded plague in the Ming Dynasty, when people would faint upon the sight of a dead rat in the street. Hence, "La Peste" ("The Plague"), a novel written by Nobel Prize winner, Albert Camus, comes easily to mind. In the novel, amidst the frenzy of the malaria outbreak, no one had any guarantee of life and no one knew his or her own fate. They were, however, sure of one thing: they had today. However, "La Peste" is after all, a novel, and therefore cannot be compared with SARS, which we encounter now.

What is the difference between SARS and other classic epidemics?

Firstly, let me go into the definition of SARS. Typical pneumonia is characterised by bacterium infection of the lungs, tissue damage, purulent, pleural effusion, trachea obstruction, collapse of lung lobes and the loss of breathing ability. Apart from the differences in the types of bacteria involved, there are differences in the aetiology of a typical pneumonia: the bacterium infects the respiratory tract in most cases and subsequently infect the lungs completely; there are fewer cases in which individual lung lobes are infected whereby the patient's condition will deteriorate more rapidly. All other types of pneumonia, which are not characterised by lung lobes infection and trachea infection, are in fact atypical pneumonia. As atypical pneumonia is associated with viruses, it is known as viral pneumonia. The commonly seen atypical pneumonia is not especially contagious, and only affects the general body functions. Thus, the present SARS epidemic is certainly very different from what we traditionally know.

Why did the WHO term the disease as "SARS"? This is probably because this epidemic is so different from the known traditional atypical pneumonia. Firstly, patients experience a lack of oxygen easily and therefore require the aid of modern respiratory equipment in order to breathe. Secondly, this syndrome can be contagious enough to infect a substantial number of people widely under some circumstances.

When the first SARS patient was warded in our department, no one knew the cause of this disease, nor were any precautions taken. As a result, over a hundred people who had been in close contact with this patient fell ill one after another. Among them were many doctors and nursing staff who had cared for this patient – therapists, medical students, medical colleagues, neighbouring patients, patients' relatives and friends, and other technicians. A visitor who had contracted this disease unknowingly transmitted the virus to other friends in a densely populated building, which eventually caused these friends to fall ill as well. The disease subsequently spread to hundreds of others residing in the building and other buildings nearby. The SARS outbreak has not only shocked the world, but is also an unprecedented epidemic outbreak in WHO's recorded history.

As the medical staff of infected hospitals are facing imminent danger of death, wouldn't they be reminded of Camus? The fact that there is no established cure for the patients who are now undergoing life-and-death struggles, is reason enough to believe that this flu outbreak is the same as the plague outbreak.

Although the mysterious causative disease agent still remains elusive since the outbreak occurred a few weeks ago, the degree of infection and its trend are unpredictable. However, apart from the elderly and other patients who are already suffering from chronic ailments, this is one disease that can be cured easily. It is strongly believed that patients will gain full recovery. Therefore, there is no need to be overly fearful of the disease.

Today, man has developed advanced technologies to solve the mysteries of life and enjoy longevity — hence resulting in a growing confidence in overcoming difficult physiological and pathological issues. It is unthinkable that this mysterious SARS outbreak has stumped many medical professionals who are struggling to contain it as well as they can, and to prevent it from worsening.

What is the real problem?

An epidemic is categorised as a public health issue, and in dealing with such an issue, we cannot depend solely on modern technology and organisational management. Although technology is an essential tool in improving public health services, substantial professional support, the initiative of the community and the participation of all citizens are required to effectively implement public health policies. This epidemic has different courses of development. If the academic, professional and community elements of public health policies can be appropriately implemented at various stages, citizens will develop an enhanced level of confidence and the spread of the epidemic will be retarded and subsequently contained. In certain parts of the world, there has been no comprehensive assessment of the initial outbreak and there was a general level of ignorance on the situation in neighbouring towns and cities. Relevant authorities had complacently assumed that only one hospital was affected and this had led them to make an announcement that they had already found the causative disease agent, when in actual fact they did not

3

have the slightest idea of what they were faced with. Despite the fact that clinical test results were highly non-representative, they chose to publicise new ways of testing, which has caused many members of the public to wait in vain. As a result, no proper preventive measures were taken, there were delays in preparing citizens to curb the spread of the epidemic, and precious time was lost. Louis Pasteur, being the pioneer in bacteriology, was the first to come up with the theory that three conditions are necessary for an epidemic to occur. There must be a causative agent, a medium, and both suitable internal and external environments for infection. Since these three conditions are co-related, the absence of any one of them will not cause an epidemic outbreak. As a lot of people have already contracted SARS in the community, the most urgent task now is to find a cure, curb its spread, ascertain its cause, carry out research, and develop tests. We should emphasise the need for a long-term plan, with a aim of finding a medical breakthrough in the near future. We should also bring together all citizens to promote the prevention of such a disease. Below are our brief suggestions for adopting good policies, which can be implemented during this epidemic period along the lines of public health.

1. Diagnosis and Categorisation of the Syndrome

Although we have mentioned that this is a disease that can be cured easily, we can only do so if we can diagnose it in time, and administer proper medical care. Before the actual cause can be ascertained, all diagnoses should be based primarily on clinical symptoms and using laboratory test results as a secondary basis. All new ways of testing are mere studies. We now know that high fever, shivering, cough, extreme lethargy, muscle aches, flu symptoms, diarrhoea and general malaise are symptoms of SARS. There are already reports published on the situations in Hong Kong and China which are in fact very good references for other parts of the world.

In Hong Kong, the health of a group of patients has deteriorated rapidly which has caused them to develop difficulties in breathing. Others undergo the incubation period of five to seven days before conditions gradually scale to an intolerable level. Yet another quarter has a relatively moderate condition. Specialists can categorise these patients according to the actual situation, so that proper medical care can be administered.

2. Cure for an Epidemic Syndrome

All SARS patients must be treated to the stage of full recovery so that the epidemic can be eradicated. After much hard work by the Chinese and Hong Kong authorities, the administration of specific anti-virals and the flexible use of steroids have proven to be effective cures. Besides the use of drugs, the application of modern technology of oxygen resuscitation and the use of recovered patients' serum as antibodies has, except for the elderly and patients suffering from other chronic illnesses, raised the recovery percentage to more than 95%. With an assured remedy in hand, and with professional diagnostic tests, they can be logically categorised in accordance with their conditions. Those very ill and elderly patients should be warded in a well-equipped hospital. Those who are suffering from mild physical syndromes can be cared for in an ordinary hospital. For patients who fall into neither of the above two categories, they should be dealt with appropriately. During the peak of the epidemic in Hong Kong, all patients, regardless of their conditions, were sent to one particular hospital, which eventually led to a serious shortage of hospital beds. The relevant authority then realised that it was not a wise move after all. Under such circumstances, where no institution can cope with such a sudden outbreak, patient categorisation procedures should be seriously considered as part of the measures in dealing with the epidemic. In fact, epidemic hospitals in Bangladesh, which often need to handle large numbers of cholera patients, will immediately segregate their medical facilities into "suspected cases zone", "confirmed cases zone", "special care cases zone" and "recovery zone" during an outbreak.

3. Sparing No Effort in Preventing Its Spread

The government should, for example, carry out preventive checks, initiate mandatory quarantine, and conduct arrival and departure health checks. In the community, all citizens should participate in the disease prevention drive. All governmental actions are only effective in the initial outbreak period. Once the disease has spread to the entire community, the participation of all citizens becomes crucial. Once there is cooperative public awareness and participation, the healthy community will not be fearful, and citizens will understand the importance of taking care of themselves as well as others. Time is of utmost importance in curbing the spread of the disease, and before this can be accomplished, a medical remedy is still of paramount importance. Front-line medical staff are not only required to maintain the disease-preventive functions of hospitals, they also need to shoulder the heavy responsibility of controlling the spread of the disease. In summary, we should not neglect the above-mentioned work of diagnosing and patient categorisation.

4. Finding the Source and Eradicating It Completely

During this time, we can certainly collect a lot of information and data on the possible causative source, medium and how the disease can infect human beings on such a scale. After this, we can bring together the efforts of academicians, professionals, government officials and citizens in order to ascertain the source of this epidemic before developing more effective remedies and preventive measures against another outbreak. If we were to just focus on the source of this disease at the peak period of the outbreak, it will just be an act of deceiving ourselves as well as others. Under normal circumstances, research work on epidemics is not only difficult, but also requires much time. Since the outbreak of SARS, there have been three different findings. China has consistently seen the presence of Chlamydia, while Hong Kong and one German laboratory found the Paramyxovirus instead. Another academic institution, on the other hand, cultured the coronavirus and this successful test received the support of American laboratories. With these findings, we now know the complexity involved in this epidemic, which involves extraordinary bacterium and viruses, be they unigerminal, bigerminal or multigerminal. The recent surreptitious and extraordinary hypothesis is that this epidemic is caused by a mutated animal virus. Clinical research has shown that the characteristics of a disease spread can be just as highly unascertainable as its causative source. However, with the advent in the life sciences and through the cooperation of many countries, we should be able to determine its cause very soon. Despite this, some time is still needed for such work to be carried out. China's Epidemic Prevention Authority has established a three-step procedure in ascertaining the source of the disease. The virus has to be first identified. This is followed by preliminary verification of the virus using antibodies developed from patient's serum and the re-establishment of test models on animals, so that all information can be proven authentic. This is the most practical way to gradually ascertain the cause. Such work will prevent any inappropriate and over-optimistic assumptions being made during an epidemic.

5. Reformulating Public Health Policies

To reformulate public health policies is not limited to disease prevention in certain areas and hospital management, globalisation and other perspectives must be incorporated. Our standard of living and material well-being has improved. This, together with medical advancement, will minimise the threats from traditional epidemics such as cholera and flu. Except for some cities, most regions and counties have already reduced or nearly closed all large epidemic medical facilities. In Hong Kong, such a hospital had been closed for over twenty years. In fact, even if it were still in operation today, it would not have the necessary facilities to cope with this disease. From this particular epidemic outbreak, medical management teams and professionals should thoroughly understand that the most successful, systematic and advanced hospital management norms are very different from those in public health management that should be carried out in times of an epidemic crisis. If corrective actions are not implemented in time, the consequences will be unthinkable. If the epidemic preventive work is not properly carried out, medical staff will fall ill alongside other SARS patients, and this will certainly be an ironical and regrettable situation. Besides preparing to cope with large-scale disasters such as fires, air crashes, earthquakes and formulating procedures to handle a substantial number of casualties, all general hospitals should also be prepared to handle an epidemic outbreak, and the resultant infection of medical staff and of crippling hospital operation, and to actively carry out work to curb the spread of the disease. A mistake made today is the best reference for tomorrow. We need to draw up a set of procedures which will involve the participation of all citizens. Just as every household was asked to make vinegar in the province of Guangdong, China, wearing facemasks in Hong Kong has become a symbol of people mobilisation. Such an approach can be further improved upon in future.

Today, as air travel becomes more and more common, geographical borders become an ineffective controlling tool from the public health point of view. The spread of SARS through air travel has highlighted this fact. If neighbouring cities such as Guangdong and Hong Kong do not provide institutional support and show humanitarian care for each other, not only will people of these two regions suffer, but others will also be harmed. We hope to put into practice health and disease-prevention joint management procedures when we are faced with a crisis. SARS has spread from China and Asia to other continents. According to reports, residents of other developed countries have become resentful towards Asians and have criticised the unhygienic lifestyle of the Chinese and Asians that could have possibly caused such an outbreak to spread to the other parts of the world. We must admit that a dense population and an undesirable living environment in China and many parts of Asia are the best breeding grounds for an epidemic. Infectious diseases, which continue to strike less-developed regions, are a rare sight in developed countries. However, is the present outbreak really caused by an unhygienic and dirty living environment?

Many years ago, microbiologists have warned that the use of antibiotics is an illogical remedy. This is because there are far too many types of antibiotics and the choice of antibiotics as well as its dosage is not prescribed with discretion. This has seriously tipped the biological balance of bacterium and microorganisms, and has subsequently led to the breeding of new diseases and diseases which are never known to man. To date, we have yet to ascertain the cause of this mysterious SARS outbreak. Could it be caused by any of the microorganisms? Could this be the specific effect of using antibiotics? Are highly populated and unhygienic developing countries the culprits then? Or are they the victims?

In this era of globalisation, a modern epidemic outbreak concerns everyone in the world and it is no longer an issue that is confined to a hospital, a city, a region or a continent. Although it has originated from China today, and has spread to Asia, it may come from America tomorrow. No country or region can be a complacent bystander during a global epidemic outbreak. Only when we have shared information and ascertained its source, researched its cause, and discussed medical cures and other areas jointly, can we then have the opportunity to curb such a disease.

Two years ago, the Ebola virus in mid-Africa afflicted 3000 people, leaving more than 500 dead. Today's SARS is not as deadly as the Ebola virus, but it continues to infect many parts of the world. There is no sign of it stopping in the near future. Despite being hit most badly, Asians have gained a good amount of wisdom. In China, the attitude towards handling this outbreak has changed from a passive to a pro-active one, which shows that our views and actions in coping with such a modern epidemic are becoming more and more globalised.

The world of Camus fifty years ago was so much different from our world today in terms of politics, economy, macroscopic issues and world views. Medical staff of badly-infected hospitals are seeing colleagues falling ill one after another, and increasingly more new infected patients are being warded. Their feeling of helplessness and fear is similar to that of the doctors described in Camus' novel. Life is fragile, and there is certainly no guarantee of living through today. Knowledge, technology, personal abilities, and rules and regulations cannot provide us sufficient protection at all. The restraints of such rules and regulations also hinder our fight for survival, which Camus mentioned in his novel. That is the reason why he wrote, "In times of epidemic, there is no hero or saint." Despite the fact that non-medical members of the public have expressed gratitude and respect towards medical professionals, those who are in the field of medical care know too well the feeling of helplessness under such a precarious environment. Regardless of changes in the environment, the strong belief in fighting for survival, and the will to live on, will not diminish after Camus' era. What all medical practitioners strive to achieve is to first ensure their survival before trying their best to assist others to live on.

Political leaders should analyse the cause, effect, gains and losses when formulating and implementing policies. Specialists should carry out a substantial amount of research so as to produce valuable academic papers. However, they should never forget what others have gone through, the events that have happened, the factors that rule changes, and those who were hurt or rescued. These memories will linger in our minds for a long time.

Camus had poked fun at the medical profession. He had purposely allowed a hero in his novel to contract the disease and subsequently die just when the outbreak was contained. Another character became insane amidst celebrations. He also prophesised that the containment of the disease did not mean total eradication. It would only represent the hibernation of the disease, which would strike again when the appropriate time comes. Modern diseases cease to hide in some dark corners anymore. They have not, in the process of continuous human destruction of the environment that is fuelled by greed and selfishness, stopped mutating into even more mysterious and deadly diseases and causative agents, and will not cease to attack human beings. The tranquility which we will experience after an epidemic outbreak is never real. When we have obtained much new medical knowledge and skills, we will often forget the epidemic of survival that has already caused irreversible destruction to our long-desired peace and tranquility.

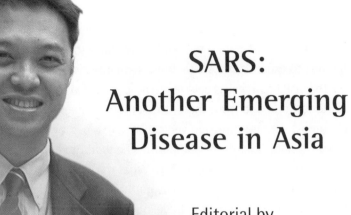

SARS:
Another Emerging
Disease in Asia

Editorial by
Dr Ooi Eng Eong

Dr Ooi Eng Eong MBBS, MSc (Medical Microbiology), DLSHTM,
PhD is Head of the Environmental Health Institute, National
Environment Agency, research interests include epidemiology
of dengue and other flaviviruses in Singapore, and dengue
prevention and control.

As this book goes to print, health authorities in many countries are still figuring out
how to contain the spread of this new respiratory illness that has been officially
called severe acute respiratory syndrome (SARS). This is not the first time east and
southeast Asia has been hit by infectious disease that left a trail of devastation. In
the last half-a-decade alone, we have witnessed several outbreaks, such as bird flu
(H5N1 influenza) in Hong Kong in 1996 to 1997; human enterovirus 71 in Malaysia,
Taiwan and Singapore in 1997, 1998 and 2000, respectively; as well as Nipah virus
in Malaysia and Singapore in 1998 to 1999.

 The current SARS outbreak also has one striking similarity to those listed above.
All these outbreaks have no prior precedent, either in terms of the aetiological
agents or the diseases they caused. H5N1 influenza is a bird virus and until the
outbreak in Hong Kong, it was believed that bird influenza virus would not infect
humans and vice versa. Likewise, the appearance of severe respiratory and
neurological disease among pigs and pig farmers in Malaysia in 1998 saw the

identification of a novel paramyxovirus now called nipah virus. There were several outbreaks of EV71 before the one in Malaysia and Taiwan but the latter group was the first to experience a severe brain stem infection.

This SARS outbreak is believed to have started in south China, which then spread to Hong Kong and from there, to Vietnam, Singapore, Canada and many other countries. The transmission vehicle is man, aided by convenient, affordable and rapid transportation from one part of the world to another. This is also a reason why many diseases are emerging. What may be confined to a small village in a remote part of the world can now get halfway across the globe within 24 hours! With more and more people traveling by airplanes, the likelihood of such events happening again can only increase.

Current available laboratory evidence also point towards a virus, coronavirus, as the causative agent although other possibilities include a paramyxovirus and a human metapneumovirus. While most coronaviruses cause common cold and flu-like illnesses, it is believed that the coronavirus causing SARS is unlike those that we have encountered before and is likely to have crossed over to man from animals. Although this is speculative at this stage, it would not be surprising should this be proven at a later stage as many zoonotic diseases, like avian flu and the nipah virus encephalitis, are severe.

The toll of outbreaks such as SARS will not only take the form of unfortunate loss of lives and long term physical disabilities but also in terms of dollars and cents as well as social cohesiveness. The world economy is still affected by the events of 9/11 and the Bali bombing. The war in Iraq is another factor of uncertainty. Measures needed to contain the spread of SARS have limited the workforce, both through quarantine and school closures. Many are staying away from crowded places, such as shopping centres. Many of those who can put off business trips and overseas travel have done so. What would add to the tragedy would be for those who are in one way or another affected by this outbreak to be ostracised by their community. In Singapore, a seven-month pregnant nurse was asked to use the stairs instead of an elevator to return to her seventh floor apartment simply because she tends to SARS patients. Some bus and taxi drivers pick up speed at the sight of a fare near the hospital dedicated to caring for SARS patients. These are signs of fear, especially that of the unknown, that may pull society apart instead of together at a time of crisis.

The primary aim of this book is thus educational. Scientific papers describing the cases, the epidemiology of the outbreak and laboratory evidence of the aetiological agent have already started making their way to press. This book is not meant to be another of such publication. Instead, it is meant to be an easy read for those who are interested in the recent events that have affected many lives. It details the course of the outbreak as well as the timing and the types of responses that were made by the various health authorities in combating the spread of this new viral disease. It also describes some simple preventive measures that can be taken to protect oneself.

While the sections describing the chronological events may appear to be history, they provide a basis for the currently prescribed disease control and prevention. In most cases, the virus is transmitted in the setting of caring for the sick. Relatives of SARS cases as well as professional healthcare workers make up the bulk of SARS cases. This indicates that the disease is more likely to be transmitted when the patients are in the later stages of illness where hospitalisation is necessary. Should this disease be most infective in the early phase of the illness, community spread would have been the common theme. While there is a hypothetical possibility that this virus spreads before a person can be diagnosed with SARS and hence isolated, there are over a thousand SARS cases and for many of these, where and from whom they acquired the infection have been traced. Such data should be considered in the face of uncertainty raised by hypothetical possibilities. Epidemiological information should form the basis for infection control.

It is also hoped that the events recorded here, along with the subsequent understanding of the causative virus, its origin and mode of spread, will become learning points to prevent outbreaks of SARS in the future and to have disease control systems in place in the event of an outbreak happening. The responsible party is also not confined to the health authorities since the disease affects many parts of society and all parties involved, from those that deal with the economy to those that deal with social well-being, should use this outbreak as a learning opportunity.

How long this outbreak will last is anybody's guess. There are still many unknown factors, from the situation in China to the exact cause of this illness. There is, however, sufficient information to be gleaned from the outbreak thus far and I hope this book would serve to be a source of such information.

Chapter 1

INTRODUCTION

Outbreak!

On 12 March 2003, the World Health Organisation (WHO) issued a global alert on the outbreak of a new form of pneumonia-like disease. This illness, officially known as severe acute respiratory syndrome (SARS), is potentially fatal and highly contagious, and has spread quickly to many parts of the world in a matter of a few weeks. Aided by globalisation and the ease of air travel today, the disease has been reported in many countries such as China, Hong Kong, Vietnam, Singapore, Canada and the US, with a large number of infections and a significant number of deaths.

It was not too long ago that Asia experienced several new and contagious diseases such as the "bird flu"[1] and the Nipah virus disease.[2] As the agents of transmission for these two diseases were chickens and pigs respectively, the solution was relatively easy: refrain from consuming these animals and slaughter the existing livestock. Even as the spectre of these previous flu epidemics has barely been exorcised, Asia has to deal with yet another highly communicable disease — and possibly a more hazardous one at that. And because SARS is transmitted person-to-person, extermination of the agents of transmission would not be a plausible solution.

A Highly Contagious and Dangerous Disease

There are three main factors that make SARS a particularly difficult problem to deal with. First, victims who suffer from the illness display symptoms that are very much

---

[1] The outbreak of the "bird flu" was in 1997, and it was generally limited to Hong Kong.
[2] The Nipah virus wrecked havoc in Malaysia in 1999, affecting mainly agricultural workers.

similar to those of the common flu. It usually begins with a high fever (over 38°C), accompanied by symptoms such as headache, sore throat, shortness of breath and dry cough. This makes it difficult to distinguish SARS from the typical cold. Before the alert on the disease was sounded, many initial cases were wrongly diagnosed as common flu; and general practitioners sent patients home prescribing them with regular antibiotics.

The second worrying characteristic of SARS is that it spreads from person-to-person with ease. Experts have established that the illness is spread by "close contact". The virus is believed to have the resilience to survive out of the human body for a few hours. Hence, an infected person can release droplets of bodily fluids containing the virus into the air when he coughs, or when he rubs his mouth or nose and touches an object. The virus can be passed on to a second person who breathes in the droplets, or who touches a contaminated object such as a door knob and rubs his face. The ease of infection has led to a great number of people being infected at the onset of the outbreak. Investigations have shown that most of the infected are mostly family members and friends of the victim, or health workers.

Lastly, SARS is dangerous because with an incubation period of less than ten days, it acts fast — and in some cases, kills fast. Although its fatality rate is not exceptionally high at 4%, its high infection rate can result in a significant number of deaths. SARS is also more dangerous for older people who have weaker immune systems or are already suffering from health complications like heart problems, diabetes and high blood pressure. Most of the victims who were killed by SARS were middle-aged or older folks with inherent health problems. For this group of people, SARS has the capability to rapidly complicate their existing health problems and cause their physical conditions to deteriorate rapidly. However, there were also a few cases whereby fit and young adults fell ill quickly and had to breathe with the aid of respirators within a week of infection.

An infected person can release droplets of bodily fluids containing the virus into the air when he coughs, or when he rubs his mouth or nose and touches an object. The virus can be passed on to a second person who breathes in the droplets, or who touches a contaminated object such as a door knob and rubs his face.

Tracing the Origin

SARS is widely believed to have originated from Foshan – Guangzhou Province (佛山-广州) of China at the end of last year. Reportedly, doctors in the Chinese province began seeing increasing numbers of patients with flu-like symptoms in November 2002. Initially, the Chinese paid no special attention to it, as Spring is a season when many people tend to fall sick due to climatic changes. However, as the conditions worsened for some patients, the authorities soon realised that they were facing a new kind of disease that the world has not seen before.

It is alleged that the authorities kept a tight lid on the matter, and passed a gag order on the media. The Guangdong government even made a public statement in mid-February saying that the spread of the illness has been brought under control.

The Spread

However, the disease soon found its way to Hong Kong, and subsequently, to more than 20 countries in the rest of the world. According to investigations carried out by Hong Kong authorities, the territory's first "index case"[3] was a 64-year-old doctor from China who had treated SARS patients in Guangzhou. The doctor, who stayed at the Metropole Hotel in Monk Kok on 21 February 2003, was admitted to hospital with SARS symptoms on the next day, where he died on 4 March 2003. It was later discovered that five other guests of the hotel who had stayed on the same floor as the doctor (the ninth floor) also contracted the disease. Three of these guests were female tourists from Singapore while the other two were Canadians.

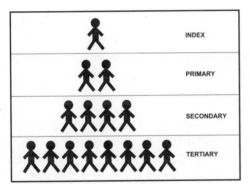

Pyramid of Infection *The source viral carrier is known as the "index" case. A person infected by the index case is referred as a "primary" case. Subsequent tiers of infection are known as "secondary" and "tertiary" cases.*

Experts think that it is highly probable that six of the guests from the hotel

---

[3] An index case refers to the source of the infection in a particular region. Refer to the figure for a graphical representation of the "pyramid of infection".

contracted the disease from the doctor, who brought the virus into Hong Kong from mainland China. It was speculated that the seven persons must have been in close proximity with one another at some point of time, such as in at a lift lobby or in an elevator. The virus could have been passed to the others when the doctor coughed or sneezed.

A Hong Konger who visited a friend at the hotel during the doctor's stay also came down with the disease. The 26-year-old man subsequently spread the disease to dozens of medical and non-medical staff of the Prince of Wales Hospital where he was warded. This hospital is perhaps the institution that is most badly hit by the illness due to the authority's initial unawareness of it. An alarming 60% of the hospital staff, including the Chief Executive of the hospital, have become infected. Similarly, a number of hospital staff in Vietnam, Singapore and Canada have also come down with the illness. The fact that hospital staff need to be in "close contact" with infected patients puts them at higher risk. After the method of viral transmission became clearer, hospitals are taking preventive measures such as making their staff wear gloves, masks and gowns; and taking extra care to isolate infected patients.

In Hanoi, Vietnam, a 48-year-old businessman from the US fell ill and was admitted to the French Hospital on 26 February 2003. He had travelled to Hong Kong and China before arriving in Vietnam. Shortly after that, an outbreak occurred in Vietnam, whereby many hospital staff became infected. The businessman later succumbed to the disease and died. Although the Vietnam authorities described the disease as under control, there has not been much media coverage on the situation in Vietnam to verify this.

The outbreak in Singapore is believed to have been caused by the three women who were infected in the Metropole Hotel in Hong Kong. After returning to their home country, all three of them fell ill, were hospitalised and were found to have contracted SARS. This was not before they had unknowingly spread the illness to many people with whom they came into contact, including several family members

Tracking the Virus

16 November 2002
Mysterious respiratory illness started in Foshan, Guandong.

11 February 2003
Provincial officials in Guangdong reported 305 cases and 5 deaths.

21 February 2003
Doctor from Guangzhou passed the disease to other hotel guests at the Metropole Hotel, Hong Kong

26 February 2003
US businessman who travelled to China and Hong Kong admitted to French Hospital in Hanoi. He was diagnosed with SARS.

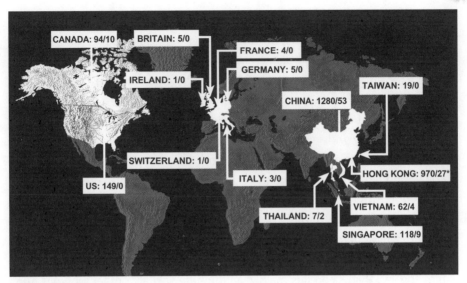

Global Outbreak *Aided by air travel, the disease spread rapidly on a global scale.*
Key: Country: Number of infections/ Number of deaths
(Figures correct as of 9 Apr 2003)

and friends. By the end of March 2003, the island-state had more than 80 cases of infection and four deaths.

The SARS cases in Canada are linked to the two Canadian tourists who stayed at the Metropole Hotel in Hong Kong. Similar to what happened in Singapore, the disease was brought back to their home countries when they returned. Ontario was most badly affected, while British Columbia saw a couple of cases. By the end of March 2003, the former had more than 40 cases of infection while the latter witnessed 2 cases. Both of the source patients later succumbed to the illness and died.

By mid-March 2003, reports of SARS cases were reported in many other countries such as US, Taiwan, Thailand and several European countries. Initial investigations revealed that all the outbreaks had origins in Asia. The viral carrier, when that could be traced, was almost always someone who had made a recent trip to China, Hong

5 March 2003
An elderly Canadian woman died in Toronto after a recent visit to Hong Kong.

12 March 2003
WHO sounded a worldwide alert on SARS.

13 March 2003
Singapore reported that 3 cases in people who have recently visited Hong Kong.

18 March 2003
Several countries in Europe report cases of SARS.

End-March 2003
40+ cases in Canada; 800+ cases in China; 500+ cases in Hong Kong; 90+ cases in Singapore; 50+ cases in US; 50+ cases in Vietnam.

Kong, Vietnam or countries in the Asia region.

The disease spread extremely swiftly. By the end of March 2003, it has infected more than 1500 people and claimed more than 50 lives globally.

The rate and ease with which SARS spread has alarmed the WHO and governments, and caused much concern, paranoia and even fear among the populace in countries that are most severely affected. As the number of infected cases rises steadily with every passing day, governments implement emergency measures to contain the disease while scientists and doctors work frantically in hospitals and labs in order to find the cause — and hopefully a cure — for it.

Although SARS has not yet developed into a pandemic, some health experts have likened this outbreak to the initial emergence of the Acquired Immune Deficiency Syndrome (AIDS) epidemic in the 1970s when health experts struggled to identify the symptoms and cause of the disease. However, one notable difference is that the AIDS virus spreads mainly via intimate sexual contact whereas SARS spreads through mere close contact. This could imply that unless properly contained, the disease might spread like a wildfire, given its apparent ease of infection.

Containment

In Hong Kong, Singapore, Canada and the US, the authorities were able to trace the outbreak by back-tracking the routes of the victims. This is extremely important, as it would be on this basis that the government can take action and implement various measures to curb the spread. The investigations in these countries were also quite open and transparent, and the media generally has access to much of the investigation results, which in turn, are disseminated to the public.

China's initial relative governmental silence on the SARS outbreak within its borders means that the media — and the world — know little about the actual situation in the country. On 26 March 2003, the authorities in mainland China suddenly announced that 792 people in China were infected with SARS with a death toll of 34.[4] The Chinese publicly admitted the seriousness of the situation, and openly asked for assistance and support from the WHO. The organisation immediately dispatched a team of experts to the country to help China contain the disease and also to study it.

---

[4] These figures reflect the official number of cases only up to the end of February 2003. China has said that it is unable to provide daily up-to-date figures.

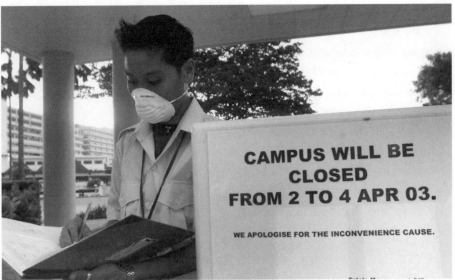

School Suspended *This polytechnic in Singapore was closed after a student was found to be infected with SARS.*

Realising the severity of the threat posed by SARS, governments began to take preventive measures to isolate patients, educate the public about the disease, and implement preventive policies in attempts to contain it.

Singapore was the first country in Asia to take decisive actions to tackle this public health threat. On 26 March 2003, the Republic announced the drastic measure of closing all its public schools, from Primary Schools up to Junior Colleges for nearly two weeks. It also invoked the Infectious Disease Act, under which all the people who have come into contact with infected victims have to be quarantined.

Taking the cue from Singapore, Hong Kong also announced the closure of its public schools the next day, and used its own legislative means to enforce the quarantine of suspected cases. When about 200 cases of infection was detected among residents of a particular apartment, the whole building was cordoned off, with policemen (who wore protective garb including masks, gloves and gown) setting up barricades and preventing anyone from entering and leaving the building.

With the highest number of infections on the North American continent, Canada took the situation very seriously. In Ontario, the authorities raised a public alert on SARS and restricted patient and visitor movements in hospitals. It also sounded a warning to discourage its citizens from visiting Asian countries that are badly affected by SARS.

Airports in some countries are also taking precautionary measures by screening their passengers, and then isolating those who are suspected of having SARS. Specially trained medical personnel are stationed at the airports, and suspected cases are either quarantined or sent directly to hospitals in ambulances. Many countries around the world have warned their citizens about the disease, and advised them to postpone or cancel any travel plans to countries like China, Hong Kong, Vietnam and Singapore.

Despite all the measures taken by various governments, no one can claim authoritatively that the disease has been contained at this point in time, as it is still premature to assess the results of the preventive measures. Many health experts are of the opinion that even if the crisis is handled well, it would take at least a few months to bring the disease under control.

Impact and Ramifications

SARS emerged at a time when the world is experiencing much economic and socio-political turmoil. Many countries around the world, especially those in Southeast Asia, are still struggling to pull themselves out of a global economic recession. The shock and horror of the September 11 terrorist attack on the US is still fresh on the minds of many people. With the heightened religious tensions brought about by Al

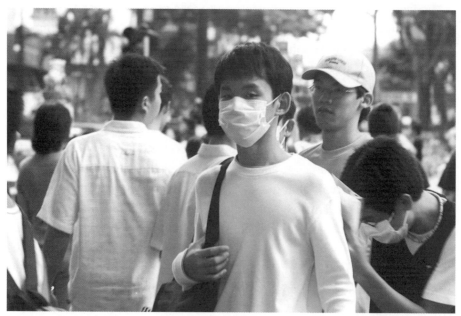

Masked! Face masks quickly became sold out as more and more people take personal preventive measures.

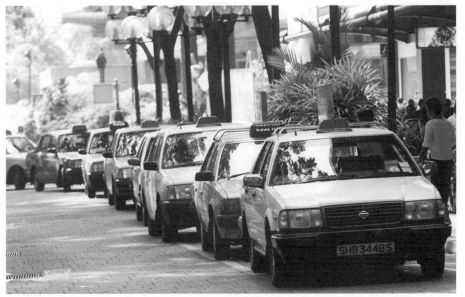

Taxi Queue *Empty taxis line up at a cab stand in downtown Singapore as Singaporeans refrain from taking taxis.*

Qaeda's clandestine terrorist operations, the world is shrouded in a cloud of insecurity. Political and economic uncertainties were again increased considerably when the US-Iraq standoff escalated into a full-fledged war in mid-March 2003. The SARS outbreak could not come at a worse time.

The rapid rate of infection, coupled with the initial ignorance of the disease, shocked and unnerved everyone. Even when information about it surfaced slowly, thanks to the tireless efforts of medical researchers, the number of infections and deaths continued to rise steadily.

One social impact of SARS is the general paranoia that it triggered. People in badly affected places such as Guangzhou, Hanoi, Hong Kong and Singapore are shocked and worried by the disease. Many of them consciously avoid public places where lots of people congregate, such as public buses, trains, shopping centres, cinemas and swimming pools. Others went about their daily lives donning face masks. Not surprisingly, face masks were sold out in almost all the places where the disease struck. The media gave broad and regular coverage on the development of the situation, and the disease has become the most talked-about topic in society. There was also a frenzied demand for vitamins and Chinese medical herbs that supposedly strengthen a person's immune system.

The sense of paranoia among people was clearly evident when the

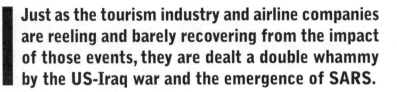

> **Just as the tourism industry and airline companies are reeling and barely recovering from the impact of those events, they are dealt a double whammy by the US-Iraq war and the emergence of SARS.**

authorities in Singapore openly searched for a cabby who had ferried an infected woman to the hospital, so as to quarantine him. The public's response to this was to play safe, and to refrain from taking taxis for fear of hopping onto the "contaminated cab". Taxi drivers complained that their business dipped by as much as 50%, and this could be attested by the long queues of taxis at cab stands all over the island.

The terrorist attacks in New York and Bali in the past two years dealt a big blow to global tourism and air travel. Just as the tourism industry and airline companies are reeling and barely recovering from the impact of those events, they are dealt a double whammy by the US-Iraq war and the emergence of SARS.

Many countries in Southeast Asia rely heavily on tourism. The Singapore and Hong Kong tourism industries account for 10% and 7% of their GDPs respectively. With the global warning by the WHO and various governments against travelling to Hong Kong, China, Vietnam and Singapore, these countries are bound to experience a significant drop in the number of visitors. A drop in the number of tourists would certainly affect related industries like hotelling, F&B (food and beverage), retail and entertainment. Already, shopkeepers in Hong Kong are complaining of dramatic drops in sales volume since the outbreak of SARS. Airlines and hotels in these countries also received numerous cancellations as people put off their travel plans. The number of flights to the affected countries has been reduced in order to cut costs for airline companies. The loss of tourist dollars and the self-imposed quarantine of some people certainly does not augur well for retailers.

Some companies were directly affected by the disease when their employees became infected by SARS. So far, two major companies — Hewlett Packard (HP) and Motorola — have discovered cases of SARS infection among their workers. In Hong Kong, one employee of HP was suspected to have contracted the disease after developing SARS symptoms. The management of HP immediately shut down its 300-person, 5-storey office and engaged professionals to clean and disinfect the office. In Singapore, mobile phone maker Motorola Inc. pulled an entire shift out of operation in its Ang Mo Kio plant after one of its night shift workers had contracted SARS.

Both Hong Kong and Singapore suspended their public schools for about two weeks. Although relieved by the precautionary measure, parents and teachers have expressed concerns about how this will affect the children's academic work and impending tests and examinations. The school children's reaction seems to be more nonchalant; many seem oblivious to the risks posed by the disease, as throngs of teenagers could be spotted hanging out at shopping centres in Singapore after the nation-wide closure of schools.

Identifying the Virus and Searching for a Cure

As doctors in hospitals fought to save infected patients, scientists and epidemiologists worked overtime in their research labs in an attempt to identify the cause and the cure.

Scientists from the Chinese University of Hong Kong and the Prince of Wales Hospital have pinpointed the cause of this mysterious respiratory illness to that of viral origin. By examining extracted tissue samples from SARS infected patients and analysing them, the virus was initially believed to belong to the paramyxoviridae family. However, further studies have shown that it is more likely to be a type of coronavirus. This finding is congruent with research results in Germany, the US and Singapore. The researchers estimate the incubation period of the virus to be between three to seven days. This has prompted authorities to impose "10-day quarantines" for suspected cases. From case studies made so far, it is thought that the disease only becomes highly contagious after the infected person develops symptoms of the disease. Also, the experts believe that the virus is rather hardy, and is capable of surviving for a few hours outside the host body.

As coronaviruses are generally not fatal, experts believe that the variant that causes SARS is probably a new mutation of existing strains. Thus, scientists are still working to identify the virus and its characteristics so as to develop an accurate test to confirm infection; and to find a cure and vaccine to combat it.

Currently, doctors who are treating the patients are having limited success using a combination of antiviral drugs that are meant for other forms of coronaviruses and steroids. Hong Kong doctors recently also reported promising results when using the serum of patients who have recovered to treat infected patients. However, it is premature to celebrate, as the effectiveness of these methods is still limited and needs further testing — a foolproof cure has yet been discovered.

And because of that, the battle against SARS is still ongoing, and experts are saying they are not seeing the light at the end of the tunnel yet. It will probably be a long battle that will lead to substantial social and economic repercussions. It will be a battle that will see many casualties even if we triumph in the end. We are fighting only to minimise casualties and to avoid an epidemic of a global scale that could decimate populations and produce catastrophic results.

Chapter 2

FLU'S FURY
Warning from History

An epidemic is defined as an outbreak of a contagious disease that spreads rapidly and widely, infecting many individuals in an area or a population at the same time. The bird flu, Nipah virus and severe acute respiratory syndrome (SARS) outbreaks were such epidemics that had caused health scares in many parts of the world, particularly in the Asian region.

Bird Flu

Influenza Viruses

There are altogether three main types of influenza virus — types A, B and C. The first two types infect *Homo sapiens* (humans) and cause disease epidemics almost every year, while the third type causes a mild respiratory illness and are not thought to cause epidemics.

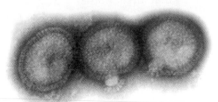

The influenza virus

Influenza type A viruses are further classified into subtypes based on two proteins on the surface of the virus. These proteins are called haemagglutinin (H) and neuraminidase (N). The current subtypes of influenza A viruses found in people are A(H1N1) and A(H3N2). Influenza types A(H1N1), A(H3N2) and B strains are included in influenza vaccines, which do not protect against type C influenza.

> The influenza type A(H5N1) virus has the ability to change itself, becoming resistant or even immune to vaccines as it spreads. Although still relatively inefficient at this point, this strain is thought to be able to mutate to the form when it becomes capable of both bird-to-human and human-to-human transmissions.

The flu virus is made up of eight RNA segments that code for at least ten proteins. Its RNA can reassort easily when two viruses (even from different host species) infect the same cell. In the case of type A viruses, their cell-surface proteins can cause epidemics when they mutate in ways that permit them to evade the host immune system.

Influenza viruses can change in two different ways, namely *antigenic drift* and *antigenic shift*. In antigenic drift, small changes continually occur in the virus over time, resulting in new virus strains that may not be recognised by the body's immune system. In antigenic shift, an abrupt, major change occurs in the type A viruses, resulting in new haemagglutinin and neuraminidase proteins in influenza viruses that infect humans. Such a shift results in a new influenza A subtype.

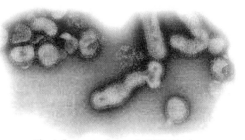

The influenza subtype A (H5N1) virus

When shift happens, most people have little or no protection against the new virus. While influenza viruses are changing by antigenic drift all the time, antigenic shift happens only occasionally. Type A viruses undergo both kinds of changes, while type B viruses change only by the more gradual process of antigenic drift.

The 1997 Bird Flu Virus

In 1997, thousands of chickens in poultry farms throughout northwestern rural Hong Kong died suddenly. Soon after, the first human cases were reported. Researchers at the virus laboratory of the Hong Kong Department of Health, aided by experts from the United States Centers for Disease Control and Prevention, Atlanta (CDC), identified the disease agent as the influenza subtype A(H5N1) virus. This

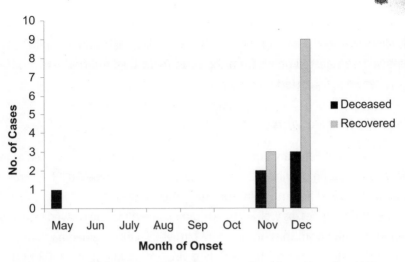

Epidemic curve of influenza type A (H5N1) cases in Hong Kong, May—Dec 1997
(Source: modified from Hong Kong Health Department)

potentially deadly strain of virus evolved from an antigenic shift-type mutation of the original influenza type A virus.

Previously known only to exist in poultry, the type A(H5N1) virus was first noticed in a three-year-old boy who later died in Hong Kong from ailments including pneumonia, inflammation of the brain, respiratory disease and Reye syndrome*.

The influenza type A(H5N1) virus has the ability to change itself, becoming resistant or even immune to vaccines as it spreads. Although still relatively inefficient at this point, this strain is thought to be able to mutate to the form when it becomes capable of both bird-to-human and human-to-human transmissions. The virus could gain this ability either by adapting itself through genetic mutations once inside the body, or by mixing with a widely circulating human flu strain, such as the type A (H3N2), in someone infected with both viruses.

International experts said that similar viruses in the past had crossed over from animal species, including birds and pigs. Spreading rapidly among humans, who have no immunity to them, they can lead to pandemics.

Vaccine development against flu strains is an extremely tricky and complicated process due to the constantly evolving nature of the virus. Flu vaccines are normally

---

* The Reye syndrome, involving the central nervous system and the liver, is a rare complication in children who may have ingested salicylates (i.e. Aspirin); it occurs mainly in children with influenza type B and less frequently in children with influenza type A or chickenpox.

produced by injecting viruses into hens' eggs and letting them multiply as the embryo develops. But in the case of the type A(H5N1) virus, being an avian flu, it kills chick embryos, so selected genes from the virus are instead inserted into a different flu virus before it is injected into the eggs.

The 2003 Bird Flu Virus

The most recent February 2003 bird flu virus outbreak that has claimed at least one life in Guangdong province, China, is also an influenza type A(H5N1) virus, though of a genetically different strain from the 1997 version.

Six internal genes, as well as the neuraminidase gene, are derived from a different genetic lineage from that of the 1997 bird virus. Only the haemagglutinin derives from the same lineage as the 1997 bird virus. In addition, the 2003 bird virus has not reassorted with a human influenza virus, which means that most likely it cannot be efficiently transmitted from human to human.

Tracing the History of Flu Outbreaks

During the last century, there have been three cases of flu pandemics:

- *Spanish Flu (1918–1919)*: Caused by the virulent organism, influenza type A (H1N1), which is known to have avian lineages. It reportedly killed more than half a million people in the United States and as many as 20–50 million people worldwide, comparable to the number of deaths in World War I. This is the highest number of known flu deaths caused by one single epidemic. Most of the people who died succumbed to the virus within the first few days of infection and the others died of complications soon thereafter. The Spanish flu was unique because almost half of the people who died were young, healthy adults.

- *Asian Flu (1957–1958)*: Over one million worldwide succumbed to the influenza type A(H2N2) virus. The Asian flu was first identified in late February 1957 in China and spread to as far as the United States four months later.

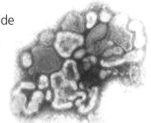

The swine flu virus

- *Hong Kong Flu (1968–1969)*: This epidemic influenza type A(H3N2) virus resulted in an international death toll of 700,000. It was first detected in Hong Kong in early 1968 and spread to the United States later that year. Such viruses are still active and circulating today.

The more recent flu outbreaks did not result in pandemics, but nevertheless still caused significant loss of human lives:

- *Swine Flu (1976)*: Soldiers at Fort Dix in New Jersey were among the first to be infected by the new swine flu virus — influenza type A(H1N1).

  Flu experts warned of a possible outbreak of epidemic proportions if the virus was not contained. It turned out to be a false alarm as the virus did not spread and a pandemic never began. However, as a result of the scare, more than 40 million Americans were vaccinated.

- *Avian Flu (1997)*: Also known as the "Bird Flu" (as detailed above), this disease resulted in the deaths of six people (a total of 18 were infected).

  The disease-causing agent, the influenza type A(H5N1) virus, is originally found only in birds. The outbreak had spurred the Hong Kong government to order the slaughter of millions chickens, as chickens were widely infected by the virus.

  Studies found that this H5N1 flu spread from poultry to people but not easily from person to person. No new human cases have been found since its eradication.

- *Influenza Type A(H9N2) Virus (1999)*: The Hong Kong Department of Health isolated influenza A viruses from two children (one- and four years of age), who were then sent to the National Institute for Medical Research (London) and the CDC (Atlanta) for identification. Both laboratories found the virus to be influenza type A(H9N2), thus marking the first confirmed human infections with viruses of this group.

  Influenza type A(H9N2) viruses usually only infects birds. It is not known how the two children in Hong Kong became infected; though both have since fully recovered. Other human type A(H9N2) infections were reported from China but no new infections have been reported since April 1999.

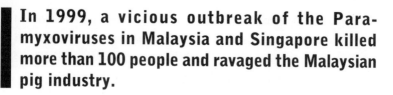

In 1999, a vicious outbreak of the Paramyxoviruses in Malaysia and Singapore killed more than 100 people and ravaged the Malaysian pig industry.

NIPAH VIRUS

In 1999, a vicious outbreak of the Paramyxoviruses in Malaysia and Singapore killed more than 100 people and ravaged the Malaysian pig industry. The causal agent was later found to be the Nipah virus (named after the location in Malaysia where it was first detected) — a newly recognised zoonotic virus. A member of the same family, called Hendra (isolated from sick horses), killed two people in Australia in 1994.

It is believed that certain species of fruit bats are a natural reservoir for both the Nipah and Hendra viruses. They are distributed across an area encompassing northern, eastern and southeastern parts of Australia, Indonesia, Malaysia, the Philippines and some of the Pacific Islands. The bats appear to be susceptible to

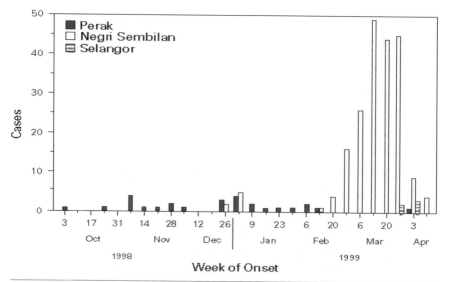

Number of cases of Nipah virus infection, by week of illness onset — Perak, Negri Sembilan and Selangor states, Malaysia 1998-1999

(*Source: Morbidity and Mortality Weekly Report, Centers for Disease Control and Prevention, Atlanta, USA*)

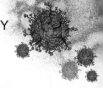

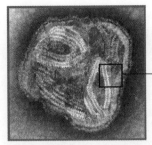

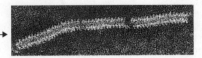

Transmission electron microscopy and negative staining reveal the "herring-bone" appearance of the helical ribonucleoprotein capsid

The human paramyxovirus virus

infection with these viruses, but do not themselves become ill. It is not clear how the virus is transmitted from bats to animals, with pigs being the most susceptible. Humans are likely to contract the virus after having direct contact with infected pigs.

The family of paramyxoviridae contains viruses that induce a wide range of distinct clinical illnesses in humans. These include the measles virus, which in rare instances is followed by subacute sclerosing panencephalitis (SSPE); mumps virus, which has symptoms of parotitis, orchitis and encephalitis; and the parainfluenza viruses which are respiratory pathogens.

Although members of this group of viruses have only caused a few focal outbreaks, the biological property of these viruses to infect a wide range of hosts and to produce a disease causing significant mortality in humans has made this emerging viral infection a public health concern.

SARS

The first suspect behind the fatal SARS disease, as discovered by Hong Kong and German researchers, was that of the Paramyxoviridae family of viruses — a group that has caused deadly outbreaks in Australia and Southeast Asia in recent years. However, the more recent research findings seem to identify the causative disease agent as a member of the Coronavirus family.

It was initially thought that the SARS epidemic might be linked to a small outbreak

The more recent research findings seem to identify the causative disease agent as a member of the Coronavirus family.

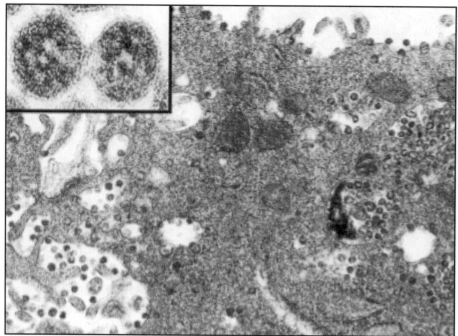

Thin section electron micrograph of infected Vero E6 cell, showing coronavirus particles within cytoplasmic membrane-bound vacuoles and the cisternae of the rough endoplasmic reticulum.
(*Source: Morbidity and Mortality Weekly Report, Centers for Disease Control and Prevention, Atlanta, USA*)

of a virulent bird flu strain called influenza type A(H5N1) in Hong Kong in February 2003. But no conclusive link has been found.

Another recent outbreak with similar symptoms, which infected over 300 people and killed five between November 2002 and February 2003 in the southern Chinese province of Guangdong, was believed to be related to the SARS outbreak. However, instead of a virus, a bacterium called *Chlamydia pneumoniae* was isolated from two of the now deceased patients. It is still unclear whether that microbe was indeed the culprit responsible.

SARS is a type of atypical pneumonia, which is usually caused by viruses, such as influenza viruses, adenoviruses and other respiratory viruses. Atypical pneumonia can also be caused by microorganisms such as Mycoplasma, Chlamydia and Legionella (which caused the deaths of 34 people worldwide from Legionnaire's disease).

Although SARS has a relatively low mortality rate — less than four per cent — it attacks the young and healthy as well as the old and frail. On 5 April 2003, it had claimed the life of 46-year-old Dr. Carlo Urbani, a World Health Organisation (WHO) expert on communicable diseases, who first identified the disease.

Scientists from three laboratories (the CDC, the Hong Kong Department of Health and the WHO) say SARS is most likely caused by a new virus from the family of coronaviruses. However, much laboratory work still needs to be done to pinpoint the exact characteristics of the virus, and development of a vaccine will take a few years.

The disease originated in China's southern province of Guangdong, before spreading to Hong Kong, from where it was then carried to Vietnam, Singapore and Canada. Cases have later surfaced in other places including the United States, France, Britain, Taiwan, Germany, and other countries.

Hitoshi Oshitani, the WHO coordinator for SARS, calls this "the most significant outbreak that has been spread through air travel in history". The surge in cases has raised concerns among Hong Kong health officials that SARS could be more contagious than initially believed.

Scientists say the strain likely originated from animals although it does not appear anything like any known human or animal viruses. Any association with influenza types A and B viruses, and also the type A(H5N1) bird flu virus (which jumped the species barrier and killed six people in the territory in 1997, and a man in February 2003) have been ruled out.

Coronaviruses, so called because of their spiky crown of protein globules, are generally not mortally harmful. They are a pest to livestock, and in humans are responsible for more than one-third of common cold cases. But in this case, researchers believe that the bugs have mutated into something far deadlier æ a rogue virus that triggers a killer pneumonia, now widely known as SARS.

The new coronavirus was isolated in Vero E6 cells from nasal and throat swab specimens of two patients in Thailand and Hong Kong with suspected SARS. The isolate was identified initially as a coronavirus by electron microscopy (EM). The little hooks sticking out of the viral body are the telltale characteristics that help

Hitoshi Oshitani, the WHO coordinator for SARS, calls this "the most significant outbreak that has been spread through air travel in history". The surge in cases has raised concerns among Hong Kong health officials that SARS could be more contagious than initially believed.

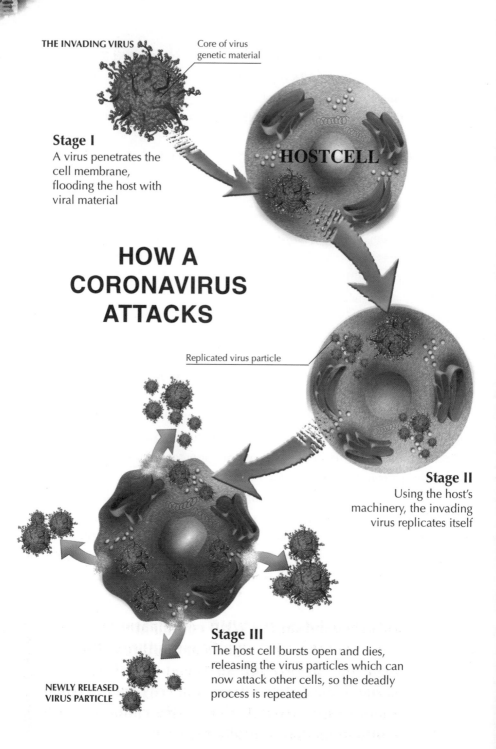

THE INVADING VIRUS

Core of virus genetic material

Stage I
A virus penetrates the cell membrane, flooding the host with viral material

HOSTCELL

HOW A CORONAVIRUS ATTACKS

Replicated virus particle

Stage II
Using the host's machinery, the invading virus replicates itself

Stage III
The host cell bursts open and dies, releasing the virus particles which can now attack other cells, so the deadly process is repeated

NEWLY RELEASED VIRUS PARTICLE

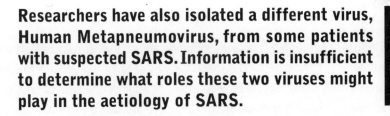

Researchers have also isolated a different virus, Human Metapneumovirus, from some patients with suspected SARS. Information is insufficient to determine what roles these two viruses might play in the aetiology of SARS.

classify the pathogens as members of the coronavirus family. The identity was corroborated by results of immunostaining, indirect immunofluorescence antibody (IFA) assays, and reverse transcriptase-polymerase chain reaction (RT-PCR) with sequencing of a segment of the polymerase gene. IFA testing of sera and RT-PCR analysis of clinical specimens from six other SARS cases were positive for the new coronavirus. Coronavirus particles were also identified by EM in cells obtained by bronchial lavage from a patient with SARS. Sequence analysis suggests that this new agent is distinct from other known coronaviruses.

To further complicate virus identification, researchers have also isolated a different virus, Human Metapneumovirus, from some patients with suspected SARS. Information is insufficient to determine what roles these two viruses might play in the aetiology of SARS. The question of whether it is an infection of one virus, a joint infection, or just coincidental infection of candidate viruses is still unanswered.

Other potential culprits in the SARS outbreak include a human parvovirus or a hantavirus (which emerged a decade ago). Most hantaviruses (spread by deer mice) are not transmitted from person to person, with the exception of the Andes virus, discovered in 1995 in southern Argentina.

Drastic steps are being taken in part because so little is known about SARS. Scientists have only begun to elucidate the viral DNA to find out its origins, how it kills and, crucially, how to counteract it. According to the WHO, the coronavirus, while it can spread quickly, is actually less contagious than the average influenza virus. But once inside a human host, it can be virulent. The pathogen causes high fever and creates an "inflammatory storm" as the body's immune system attempts to fight it off.

In order to prove beyond doubt that a candidate virus is causing SARS, "gold-standard" tests will be needed. One such test is the enzyme-linked immunosorbent assay (ELISA), which can detect antibodies produced by the patient's immune system to fight a particular virus. To date, there is some success with similar techniques and several recovering patients seem to have antibodies against the coronavirus that have been isolated.

CONCLUSION

As influenza viruses are constantly mutating and changing, it is impossible to pinpoint a range of specific types and develop a series of tailor-made cures to combat them. A newly developed vaccine may be effective against one type of virus one day, but become completely useless the next. Before we can understand the mechanism behind virus transmissibility, we must first identify the molecular changes in the different genes responsible and also carry out detailed studies on the epidemiological data of the virus.

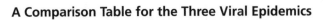

A Comparison Table for the Three Viral Epidemics

	Epidemics		
	1997 Bird Flu	**Nipah**	**SARS**
Virulent Organism	Influenza type A(H5N1) virus strain	Paramyxoviridae virus	Coronavirus
Possible Sources	Poultry (e.g. chickens, ducks, geese, etc.).	Pigs	Suspected to originate from animals (birds, chickens, ducks, etc.).
Possible Mode of Transmission	Mainly animal-to-animal. Animal-to-human transmission only through close contact with infected birds. Also possibly spread from human-to-human.	Animal-to-animal (orally) and animal-to-human possibly via close contact with contaminated tissue or body fluids of infected animals.	Spread human to human via airborne particles (>5 μm), large pathogen-laden droplet infection, or close contact with infected persons.
Symptoms	Flu-like symptoms, e.g. breathing difficulties, cold, cough, fever (above 38°C) and body aches.	Pneumotropic, affecting mainly the lungs, with high fever (above 38°C) and muscle pains (myalgia). The disease may progress to inflammation of the brain (febrile encephalitis) with drowsiness, disorientation, convulsions and coma.	High fever (above 38°C), muscle aches, sore throat and headaches; followed by pneumonia, acute respiratory distress and general malaise.
Treatment	Vaccines developed through preparation of seed virus from various H5 virus strains.	No proven drug therapies.	No known cure or vaccine. Doctors have been treating SARS patients with anti-virus drugs (e.g. Ribavarin) and steroids.
Approximated Worldwide Death Toll	Six people	Over 100 people	More than 100 people

Chapter 3

SARS TRACK
Situation Updates Around the World

Global Outbreak

Since the outbreak of SARS in early March 2003, the disease has spread rapidly to various parts of the world – a total of 17 countries in 5 continents, with the continent of Asia being the hardest-hit, followed by North America and parts of Europe. As at 7 April 2003, the cumulative number of people affected worldwide stands at 2601, with 98 cases of death. This number is expected to rise. Countries that are most severely-hit are Asian countries such as China (Guangdong Province, Hong Kong Special Administrative Region of China, Shanxi Province), Singapore and Vietnam (Hanoi), followed by Canada (Toronto) and the United States.

It was also with much regret that Dr. Carlo Urbani, an expert on communicable diseases, died on 29 March 2003 of SARS. Dr. Urbani worked in public health programmes in Cambodia, Laos and Viet Nam. He was based in Hanoi, Viet Nam. Dr. Urbani, 46 years old, was the first World Health Organisation (WHO) officer to identify the outbreak of this new disease, in an American businessman who had been admitted to a hospital in Hanoi. Because of his early detection of SARS, global surveillance was heightened and many new cases have been identified and isolated before they infected hospital staff. In Hanoi, the SARS outbreak appears to be coming under control.

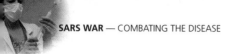

WORLD HEALTH ORGANISATION WEBSITE

Cumulative Number of Reported Cases of Severe Acute Respiratory Syndrome (SARS)

From: 1 Nov 2002 To: 7 Apr 2003

Country	Cumulative Number of Case(s)	Number of Deaths	Local Chain(s) of Transmission[2]
Australia	1	0	None
Brazil	1	0	None
Canada	90	9	Yes
China[3]	1268	53	Yes
China, Hong Kong Special Administrative Region	883	23*	Yes
China, Taiwan	21	0	Yes
France	3	0	None
Germany	5	0	None
Italy	3	0	None

Country	Cumulative Number of Case(s)	Number of Deaths	Local Chain(s) of Transmission[2]
Malaysia	1	1	None
Republic of Ireland	1	0	None
Romania	1	0	None
Singapore	106	6	Yes
Spain	1	0	None
Switzerland	1	0	None
Thailand	7	2	None
United Kingdom	5	0	None
United States	141	0	None
Vietnam	62	4	Yes
Total	**2601**	**98**	

Notes:
Cumulative number of cases includes number of deaths.

As SARS is a diagnosis of exclusion, the status of a reported case may change over time. This means that previously reported cases may be discarded after further investigation and follow-up.

1. The start of the period of surveillance has been changed to 1 November 2002 to capture cases of atypical pneumonia in China that are now recognised as being cases of SARS.

2. National public health authorities report to WHO on the areas in which local chain(s) of transmission is/are occurring. These areas are provided on the list of Affected Areas.

3. The reporting period from Guangdong Province is from 16 November 2002 to 28 February 2003.

Due to differences in the case definitions being used at a national level, probable cases are reported by all countries except the United States of America, which is reporting suspected cases under investigation.

* One death attributed to Hong Kong Special Administrative Region of China occurred in a case medically transferred from Viet Nam.

ASIA

HONG KONG

The outbreak in Hong Kong began on 11 March 2003 when health officials first recognised a cluster of cases of atypical pneumonia in the Prince of Wales Hospital. By midnight of 11 March, 50 health care workers had been screened and 23 of them were found to have febrile illness. They were admitted to the hospital for observation as a precautionary measure. In this group, eight developed early chest x-ray signs of pneumonia. Their conditions remained stable. Three other health care workers self-presented to hospitals with febrile illness and two of them had chest x-ray signs of pneumonia.

Since the outbreak on 11 March 2003, the situation in Hong Konog has been extremely critical. As of 7 April 2003, a total of 883 people have been affected, with 23 deaths. Of those affected, 208 are health care workers of Hospitals/Clinics and medical students and 675 are patients, family members and hospital visitors. Most of the medical staff affected are from the Prince of Wales Hospital.

On 1 April 2003, the Hong Kong Department of Heath announced that 213 residents of the Amoy Gardens have been admitted to hospital with suspected infection and pneumonia. On the same day, Hong Kong experienced the greatest increase in the number of infected cases, at 155. Amoy Garden is a large housing estate

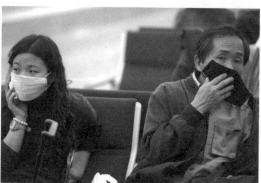
Hong Kong residents combating the SARS outbreak
(Source: Strategic Business World Monthly)

consisting of ten 35-storey blocks, where around 15,000 persons reside. It is located in Kowloon District. The Hong Kong Department of Health has issued an unprecedented isolation order to prevent the further spread of SARS. The isolation order requires residents of Block E of Amoy Garden to remain in their flats until midnight on 9 April. The decision to issue the isolation order was made following a continuing steep rise in the number of SARS cases detected in the building over the few days from 1 April. Concern about a possible outbreak in Amoy Garden mounted on 29 March 2003, when 22 of Hong Kong's 45 new SAR cases hospitalised that day were determined to be residents of the estate. On 30 March 2003, 36 of the 60 new patients admitted to hospital with probable SARS were Amoy Garden residents. Of the 213 Amoy Garden residents affected in the outbreak, 107 patients resided in Block E. In addition, most of these 107 patients from Block E live in flats that were vertically arranged. On 4 April 2003, health authorities reported investigations into sewage samples at a construction site adjacent to the Block E apartment building in Amoy Gardens, which has been the source of a large cluster of new SARS cases. A second line of investigation is concentrating on a burst sewage pipe in block E that may have epidemiological links with a visitor to Amoy Gardens, who was subsequently admitted to Hong Kong's Prince of Wales Hospital in early March and was said to have been symptomatic at the time of his visit.

Following the outbreak at Amoy Gardens, there is increasing concern about the SARS situation in Hong Kong. The continuing and significant increase in the number of SARS cases suggests that the epidemic has spread beyond the initial focus in hospitals. These developments have suggested environmental routes of transmission from a SARS infected person which may be related to contamination of common systems that link rooms or flats together. Despite the implementation of strict measures to control the outbreak, there continues to be a small number of visitors to Hong Kong who have been identified as SARS cases after their return from Hong Kong. The epidemic in Guangdong Province of China, situated adjacent to Hong Kong, is the largest outbreak of SARS reported and has also shown evidence of

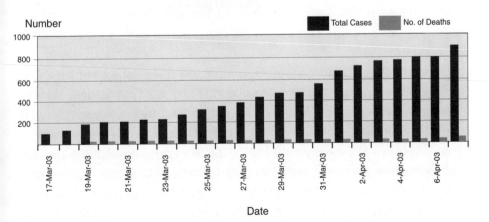

Total No. of Cases & No. of Deaths: Hong Kong

Hong Kong Department of Health website:

Latest Figures on Atypical Pneumonia
(as at 7 April 2003)

Nature	Total Admission (The numbers in bracket are those with pneumonia symptoms)
Health care workers of Hospitals/Clinics and medical students	208 (208) 69 of the patients were discharged
Patients, family members and visitors	675 (675) 58 of the patients were discharged
Total admission	833 (833) 127 were discharged 23 deaths

spread in the wider community. As a measure of precaution WHO is now recommending that persons travelling to Hong Kong and the Guangdong Province of China consider postponing all but essential trips. This temporary recommendation will be reassessed in the light of the evolution of the epidemic in the areas currently indicated, and other areas of the world could become subject to similar recommendations if the situation demands.

Earlier in March 2003, Hong Kong epidemiologists detected an unusual pattern of transmission among guests and visitors at the Metropole Hotel during the critical period of 15 to 23 February. Guests and visitors at a single floor of the hotel are thought to have spread SARS to Toronto and Singapore and to have started the outbreak in Hong Kong's Prince of Wales Hospital. No staff at the hotel have developed symptoms.

The Hong Kong Department of Health has identified the index case in the outbreak in the Prince of Wales Hospital in Hong Kong. In an outstanding example of detective work, epidemiologists have determined that seven people who contracted SARS in early March stayed in or had visited the Metropole hotel in Kowloon between 12 February and 2 March. The seven persons investigated include three visitors from Singapore, two from Canada, one mainland China visitor, and a local Hong Kong resident. The investigation revealed that all seven stayed in or visited the same floor of the hotel during the period. The local Hong Kong resident is believed to be the index case, who subsequently infected other early cases in the outbreak. He had visited an acquaintance staying at the hotel from 15 to 23 February. The visitor from Mainland China, who became sick a week before staying at the hotel, is considered the original source of the infection. No further cases have been linked to the hotel.

As of 7 April 2003, Hong Kong continued to report the largest number of new SARS cases, placing some hospitals under considerable strain. Meanwhile, a report from the Department of Health indicates that the unusual outbreak among residents in the Amoy Gardens estate, involving 268 cases, is coming to an end. Investigation of environmental samples continues at a rapid pace with support from several government departments. Evidence that the causative agent is excreted in faeces has focused attention on the possibility of an oral-faecal route of transmission, though no conclusions have been reached. The investigations have found no evidence of airborne spread.

CHINA

China remains the country with the largest number of cases. According to official reports, 1268 cases with 53 deaths have occurred as of 7 April 2003. The majority of these cases and deaths were associated with an outbreak in Guangdong Province. During that outbreak, authorities recorded 792 cases and 31 deaths from 16 November 2002 through 28 February 2003.

In mainland China, figures released by the Chinese government officials on 26 March 2003 revealed that nearly three dozens people have died and almost 800 became ill with flu-like disease. Approximately 30% of these cases are health-care workers. This greatly raises the global death toll to 51 and cumulative cases to 1, 325. On 27 March 2003, officials issued the first reports of cases and deaths in ongoing outbreaks in Beijing province and in the northern province of Shanxi. In Beijing, 10 cases and 3 deaths have occurred as of 26 March. Two of these cases involve health-care workers. In the northern province of Shanxi, four cases (with no deaths) have occurred as of 26 March. Two cases are health-care workers.

Prior to this, the Chinese authorities had said that only five people had died from a pneumonia-like illness that struck the southern Guangdong province. And for weeks, Chinese officials said only 305 people were stricken in the outbreak that started in November in Guangdong.

Total No. of Cases & No. of Deaths: China

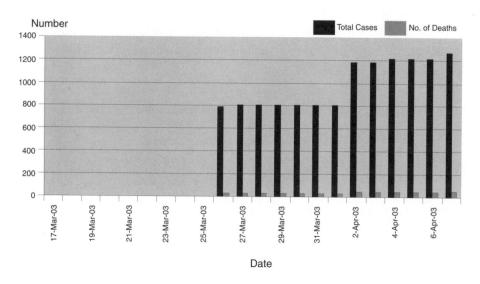

The WHO team of 5 experts arrived in Beijing on 22 March 2003 to investigate an outbreak of atypical pneumonia that began in the Guangdong Province on 16 November 2002. Experts have strongly suspected a link between the southern China outbreak and current cases of SARS that first surfaced in mid-February in Asia. The WHO investigation is being conducted in collaboration with the Chinese Ministry of Health, the Chinese Centers for Disease Control and officials from the Guangdong Province. The WHO team is expected to visit Foshan city, where the first case of SARS was reported, and Guangzhou city. The team will also visit health care facilities, review case records, and hold further discussions before returning to Beijing by 16 April 2003.

On 28 March 2003, China has further agreed to begin providing up-to-date electronic reports of SARS cases throughout China. These reports are submitted electronically as officials reports to WHO from the Ministry of Health.

In Beijing, the government of China is gearing up to fight SARS on a priority basis. Reports in the media on 3 April 2003 referred to a State Council executive meeting on SARS and described three key decisions.

- A special task force, headed by the Minister of Health Dr Zhang Wenkang, will take charge of the fight against SARS. A vice secretary-general of the State Council will coordinate actions by relevant ministries.
- The task force will provide updates on SARS to the WHO.

- A nationwide mechanism for outbreak alert and response will be set up shortly to ensure rapid detection and reporting of outbreaks.

Dr Zhang has appeared on the Chinese national TV to address SARS-related issues. The government is also holding daily press conferences. The WHO welcomes this move, which is an important way to increase awareness of the population and health-care staff of the characteristic symptoms, the need to seek prompt medical attention, and the need to manage patients according to the principles of isolation and strict infection control.

The WHO office in China has reported considerable anxiety among the international community following the death in Beijing on 6 April 2003 of a 53-year-old Finnish staff member of the International Labor Organisation. The ILO staff members were in Beijing to attend an international conference. At present it is unclear how the staff member contracted SARS. He had travelled to Beijing via Thailand, where no local transmission has been reported.

SINGAPORE

Singapore has reported the third largest number of SARS cases. As at 7 April 2003, a total of 106 people with SARS have been reported to the Ministry of Health, with 6 deaths. The total number of people who have recovered from SARS and have been discharged from hospital is 73. The remaining 31 patients are hospitalised, out of which 12 are in serious condition. The cases in Singapore are traced to the first three people who travelled to Hong Kong and contracted SARS. The disease was brought to Singapore by these three local travellers who had visited Hong Kong, where they were believed to be infected by a mainland Chinese doctor who had eventually died. The number of infected children still remains low at 3. The number of people under Home Quarantine Orders is 133.

The Ministry of Education (MOE) and Ministry of Health (MOH) have decided to close all kindergardens, primary schools, secondary schools, junior colleges and centralised institutes from 27 March to as late as 16 April. The strategy is to isolate victims and suspected cases through quarantines and restricting visits to hospitalised victims. Hefty fines will be imposed on those who break the 10-day quarantine, which was imposed under the rarely invoked Infectious Diseases Act.

SARS patients who are discharged from the Tan Tock Seng Hospital (TTSH) are

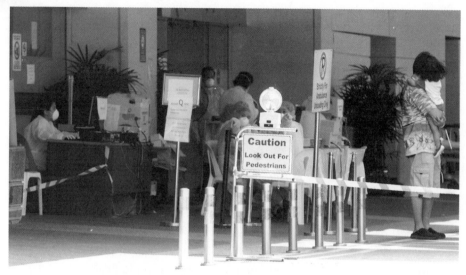

Patients screening for SARS outside Tan Tock Seng Hospital.

followed up in accordance with the guidelines from the WHO. Upon discharge, SARS patients are given medical leave for two weeks and are required to stay at home. They are reviewed by the doctors at TTSH before they return to work or school. During their two weeks' medical leave at home, their condition is monitored by staff from TTSH through daily phone calls.

On 7 April 2003, a cluster of health-care workers who are striken with SARS are reported by the Ministry of Health. A nurse from TTSH who had come into contact with a SARS patient before the patient was diagnosed with SARS was admitted on 28 Mar 2003 as a suspected SARS patient. She has since been upgraded to a probable SARS case.

Two nurses from Changi General Hospital (CGH) have been admitted to TTSH on 5 and 6 April 03 as probable SARS cases. One had close contact with a patient before she was diagnosed with SARS and was transferred to TTSH on 21 March 2003. This SARS patient was infected when she visited her sister in TTSH. At that time, a SARS patient who had yet been diagnosed was warded next to her sister at TTSH. CGH had put the whole ward staff on voluntary quarantine and the staff were followed up closely. On 2 April 2003, the nurse who had attended to the SARS patient was admitted to a single room at CGH as the clinical picture then was suggestive of dengue fever. She was later diagnosed as a probable SARS when her third chest x-ray showed changes. Her colleague who had attended to her when

Total No. of Cases & No. of Deaths: Singapore

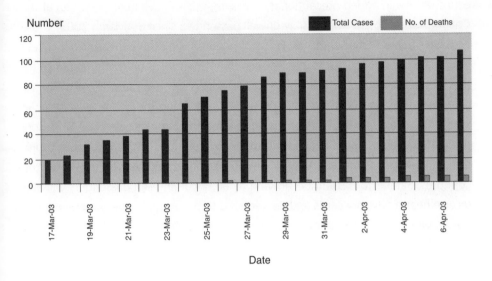

she admitted, has now been diagnosed with SARS.

A nurse from a private nursing home was admitted to CGH on 4 April 2003 for pneumonia and transferred to TTSH on 6 April 2003 for probable SARS. He is now in a serious condition in intensive care. His girlfriend, who is also a nurse at the same nursing home was admitted to TTSH on 7 April 2003 as a suspected SARS patient. Her condition has remained stable. Investigations have revealed that a resident of the nursing home was admitted to CGH on 25 March 2003 and had died of pneumonia on 30 March 2003. This nursing home resident had been earlier discharged from TTSH on 23 March 2003 for a non-SARS related condition. When the patient was in TTSH, she was warded next to a patient who was later diagnosed as a SARS case. The male nurse from the nursing home had been attending to this resident.

Arising from the transfer of staff and patients of SGH Wards 57 and 58, a total of 29 have been admitted to the SARS wards. Of these, there are four probable SARS cases (a doctor and two nurses), 18 suspected SARS cases and 7 admitted for observation. They have all remained stable.

Precautionary Measures - Air and Sea passengers:
To minimise the number of imported SARS cases, Singapore has tightened screening measures for incoming flights into the Changi International Airport from affected countries as identified by WHO. Since 18 Mar 2003, health advisory cards

51

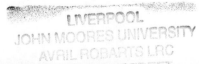

have been issued to passengers from in-bound/ out-bound flights from/ to affected countries. As an added precautionary measure, nurses have been stationed at the Changi Airport to check on visibly unwell passengers since 31 March 2003. Those who have fever will be sent to TTSH for assessment. With these measures, there are now three lines of checks for passengers on in-bound flights from affected countries – by airlines' counter staff before the passengers' boarding from these countries; crew members on board the aircraft; and nurses when the passengers arrive in Singapore. The majority of passengers from affected countries come into Singapore by air. However, as an added control, screening measures at the Singapore Cruise Centre have been tightened for incoming sea passenger vessels from affected countries. Similar to passengers arriving by air, incoming sea passengers will also receive health advisory cards and are required to go through a visual screening by nurses when they disembark. This additional measure was implemented from 3 April 2003.

HANOI, VIETNAM

In Vietnam the outbreak began with a single initial case who was hospitalised for treatment of SARS of unknown origin in late February 2003. The patient felt unwell during his journey and fell ill shortly after arrival in Hanoi from Shanghai and Hong Kong SAR, China. Following his admission to the French hospital, approximately 20 hospital staff became sick with similar symptoms.

On the 26 February 2003, the man (index case) was admitted to hospital in Hanoi with a high fever, dry cough, muscle ache and mild sore throat. Over the next four days he developed increasing breathing difficulties, severe reduction in platelets, and signs of Adult Respiratory Distress Syndrome and required ventilator support. Despite intensive therapy he died on 13 March 2003.

On 5 March 2003, seven health care workers who had cared for the index case also became ill (high fever, muscle ache, headache and less often sore throat). The onset of illness ranged from 4 to 7 days after admission of the index case.

As of 7 April 03, there have been 62 cases of SARS reported in Hanoi with 4 deaths. Thirteen of the cases are showing signs of clinical improvement. Seven people in Vietnam infected with the deadly respiratory disease been discharged from the French hospital in Hanoi. The number of cases has previously increased rapidly but then stabilised on 24 March at 58 cases, this number remaining stable for 10 consecutive days. As the maximum incubation period for SARS is thought to be 10 days, the stable number of cases over this period raised hope that Vietnam's outbreak had been brought under control. However, on 3 April a probable SARS

Total No. of Cases & No. of Deaths: Vietnam

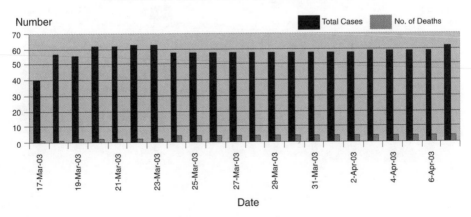

case was detected in a provincial hospital. Though the case could be linked back to the French hospital, the absence of isolation and rigorous infection control at the provincial hospital suggests that many hospital staff, patients, and visitors could have been exposed, thus possibly seeding further waves of cases. An additional three probable cases have been reported over the 3 days from 5 to 7 April 2003.

TAIWAN

Taiwan has tightened measures to prevent a SARS epidemic by declaring a city-wide alert in Taipei. As of 7 April 2003, 21 people are affected, although there are no deaths to date. This is after five employees of a major engineering company who have recently returned from China developed SARS symptoms. The city government is also tracking more than 1,000 people, including 200 or so who had boarded the same plane with the five affected employees.

The Health Department officially declared SARS a communicable disease. Anyone who defies a local health office's order to stay at home in compliance with quarantine rule would be fined up to NT$300,000. Doctors or medical institutes which fail to report any suspected cases to the Health Department or refuse to treat suspected patients will be fined NT$1 million. After the announcement, 300 people have been put under quarantine.

Public transport companies, such as subways, buses and cabs, have also started disinfecting their facilities. Jittery residents are also rushing to buy masks, driving up their prices.

Total No. of Cases & No. of Deaths: Taiwan

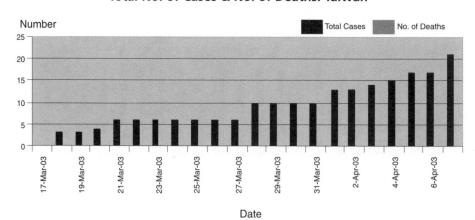

THAILAND

As of 15 March 2003, one imported case has been reported in Thailand. The case (a health care worker) travelled to Thailand on 11 March from Hanoi, Vietnam. The case is known to have had close contact with the Hanoi index case and to have been unwell on arrival in Thailand. The patient was immediately isolated on arrival in Thailand and reported to be in a stable condition and is being cared for in isolation.

On 1 April 2003, Thailand reported its second death from SARS. A Hong Kong national who was visiting relatives in Thailand died in the southern city of Haad Yai after reporting symptoms of the atypical pneumonia, a hospital official said.

As of 7 April 2003, seven people are affected with two deaths.

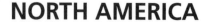

NORTH AMERICA

CANADA

As of April 7, 2003, Health Canada has received reports of 217 probable or suspected cases of SARS. There have been 9 deaths in Canada. All Canadian cases have occurred in persons who have travelled to Asia or had contact with SARS cases in the household or in a health-care setting. The largest outbreak has occurred in Ontario, where 87 probable and 92 suspected cases have been reported. British Columbia has reported 3 probable and 23 suspected cases; New Brunswick 2 suspected cases; Saskatchewan 1 suspected case; Alberta 5 suspect cases; and Prince Edward Island 4 suspected cases.

A health emergency has been declared in Toronto, Canada's largest city.

Total No. of Cases & No. of Deaths: Canada

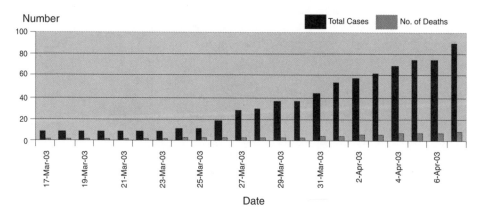

USA

In United States, a total of 141 people have also been affected by SARS, although no deaths have been reported as of 2 April 2003.

Below is a breakdown by states of the people affected from the Centers for Disease Control and Prevention (CDC) website.

Severe Acute Respiratory Syndrome: Report of Suspected Cases Under Investigation in the United States

These data were reported to the World Health Organization on April 6, 2003.

State	Suspected cases under investigation	State	Suspected cases under investigation
Alabama	1	New Hampshire	1
California	38	New Jersey	3
Colorado	5	New Mexico	1
Connecticut	2	North Carolina	5
Florida	5	New York	21
Georgia	2	Ohio	5
Hawaii	5	Oregon	1
Illinois	7	Pennsylvania	5
Kansas	1	Rhode Island	1
Maine	2	Texas	4
Massachusetts	4	Utah	5
Michigan	2	Vermont	2
Missouri	2	Virginia	2
Mississippi	1	Washington	9
Minnesota	5	Wisconsin	1
Total Suspected Cases Under Investigation			**148**

Total No. of Cases & No. of Deaths: United States

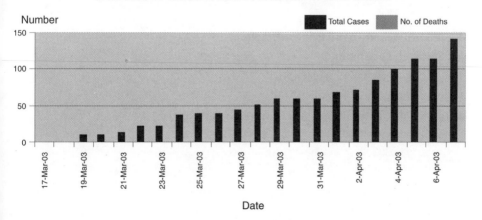

EUROPE

European countries have stepped up precautions at airports, with medical experts screening travellers - both arriving and departing - with symptoms of SARS in countries from Spain to Russia. Many governments have also issued travel advisories to citizens planning to travel to the SARS-affected region, with Belgium and Denmark becoming the latest countries to advise their citizens against travel.

As of 7 April 2003, some of the European countries affected are France, Germany, Italy, Republic of Ireland, Spain, Switzerland and United Kingdom, although no deaths have been reported. So far all the cases in Europe have been among people who recently travelled to Asia.

Switzerland has banned thousands of exhibitors from the Basel World Watch and Jewellery Fair from employing anyone who has arrived in the country from China, Hong Kong, Singapore or Vietnam since 1 March 2003. The ban affects about 5,000-7,000 employees of 350 exhibitors. As a result, some exhibitors are unable to open their stands at all because of the order.

The Dutch Health Ministry is gearing up for possible quarantine measures in case an outbreak hits the Netherlands.

German health authorities are distributing information to travellers before they board planes bound for Frankfurt airport, the biggest air hub in continental Europe. Passengers arriving in France from SARS-affected areas, including Toronto, are required to fill out forms with their contact details before leaving for their flights.

Acknowledgements

The following sources are acknowledged:
World Health Organisation
Hong Kong Department of Health
Singapore Ministry of Health
United States Center for Disease Control and Prevention

Chapter 4

WHO — SARS' MAIN FIGHTER

A Chronology of World Health Organisation's Involvement in Combating SARS

Mid February 03   Started to actively work on confirming reports of outbreaks of a severe form of pneumonia in Vietnam, Hong Kong, and Guangdong province in China. No link made between outbreaks of acute respiratory illness in Hanoi and Hong Kong and the outbreak of bird flu.

12 March 03   Issued a global alert about cases of atypical pneumonia and that the severe respiratory illness may spread to hospital staff.
In close contact with relevant national authorities and has also offered epidemiological, laboratory and clinical support.

14 March 03   Set up nine-person team to help in infection control in Hanoi.

15 March 03   Issued first SARS-related emergency travel advisory to alert national authorities and clinicians to potential cases of SARS and to urge travellers, including airline crew, with symptoms suggestive of SARS to seek medical attention. This was in response to the growing international threat posed by Severe Acute Respiratory Syndrome (SARS). Since then, WHO has conducted daily teleconferences with health authorities and WHO team members on the scene

in all areas affected by SARS. The advisory also included main symptoms and signs of SARS.

17 March 03 — WHO started to co-ordinate international effort to identify and treat SARS through its Global Outbreak Alert and Response Network. The network consists of over 150 institutions around the world. Through it, WHO has been able to get personnel to go to the field, to get guidance and advice and to gather protective equipment and other supplies within 24 hours.

Set up network of researchers from 11 leading laboratories to exchange data on a restricted web site and compare virological and clinical information during daily teleconferences.

WHO Global Outbreak Alert and Response teams in Hanoi and Hong Kong where the most new cases are presently concentrated, assist health authorities in outbreak management and in the collection of epidemiological and clinical data that can improve understanding of SARS.

18 March 03 — Set up case definitions for surveillance of SARS.

20 March 03 — Laboratories identified the Paramyxoviridae virus in specimens from patients with SARS. Set up a second network of clinicians to expedite work on diagnosis and treatment.

21 March 03 — Issued preliminary clinical description of SARS, stating its incubation period to be usually 2-7 days but may be as long as 10 days and that treatment regimens have included a variety of antibiotics to antiviral agents such as oseltamivir or ribavirin, as well as steroids.

23 March 03 — Five-person team arrived in China.

24 March 03 — Issued guidelines on the management of SARS – probable

cases, contact, contacts of probable cases and contacts of suspected cases.

25 March 03	Researchers at WHO said a paramyxovirus and a coronavirus have been identified in the tissues of patients from many different countries.
26 March 03	Organised a virtual meeting of 80 physicians from 13 localities treating SARS patients. Discussion focused on features of the disease at presentation, treatment and progression of the disease, prognostic indicators and discharge criteria.
27 March 03	Suggested affected territories, including Vietnam, Singapore, Hong Kong, Taiwan, Beijing and Guangdong province in China and Canada, to conduct simple screening procedure that included answering questions about possible symptoms that a person might have of SARS and about contacts with possible SARS cases. National authorities may also advise travellers with fever, departing on international flights from the few areas where SARS transmission has been documented, to postpone travel until they feel better. Defined close contact aboard an aircraft as sitting next to a passenger, sitting in the same row, or sitting two rows in front or two rows behind, as well as the stewardesses or flight attendants.
28 March 03	Hong Kong began using diagnostic tests for coronavirus. Tests are based on polymerase chain reaction (PCR) technology that identifies the molecular makeup of the virus thought to cause SARS. Initial studies of the tests consistently confirmed known SARS cases early in their infection and produced negative results in healthy people. Announced that China would join the global network and that the most likely agent is coronavirus.

Issued guidelines on hospital infection control and hospital discharge and follow-up policy for patients who have been diagnosed with SARS.

29 March 03   Dr Carlo Urbani of WHO, an expert on communicable diseases, died of SARS. The first WHO officer to identify the outbreak of this new disease in an American businessman, who had been admitted to a hospital in Hanoi, Dr Urbani worked in public health programs in Cambodia, Laos and Vietnam.

31 March 03   Announced possibility that SARS virus is zoonotic and may be more infectious than the Ebola virus that plagued parts of Africa.

1 April 03   Announced that some environmental factor, not the air, but perhaps water, sewage, etc., is taking this disease from one human to another. But sticks to the belief that droplet infection – person to person contact – is the major mode of transmission.

2 April 03   Issued travel advisory for travellers to Hong Kong and Guangdong province, China to consider postponing all but essential travel. This is the first time in the history of WHO that such travel advice has been issued for specific geographical areas because of an outbreak of an infectious disease.
Announced China as a full partner with WHO. With 361 new SARS cases and nine deaths in Guangdong, WHO teams went to Guangdong immediately.

4 April 03   China apologised for not doing a better job of informing people about SARS as a WHO team went to Guangdong province's Foshan where it believed the mystery illness might have first broken out.

WHO experts established preliminary agreement with those of Chinese experts that there might be more than one virus, which caused SARS.

7 April 03

A visit to the Chinese hospital in Guangdong led WHO representatives to recognise that Chinese medicine is effective for the treatment of SARS. It is especially so in reducing the length of time in which a patient is feverish and is hospitalised. Meanwhile, Shanghai has also invited WHO to help in handling and preventing SARS.

BBC said that Dr Brundtland, Director-General of WHO, had openly criticised China for not handling SARS in a timely manner.

8 April 03

While SARS diagnosis is still being made on clinical grounds and exposure only, WHO highlighted the status of currently available diagnostic tests. They are namely antibody tests, molecular tests and cell culture.

9 April 03

The WHO team of experts presented its interim report on the SARS outbreak in Guangdong province this morning to the Chinese Ministry of Health and Vice Premier Wu Yi in Beijing. The team concluded that the health system in Guangdong responded well to the outbreak, but found an urgent need to improve surveillance in the countryside. WHO signalled a concern about the warding of a large cluster of hospital staff in Singapore as potential SARS patients. Its official David Heymann said it was unusual for so many potential cases to begin on the same day if caused by contact with a patient.

Chapter 5

POLICIES AND MEASURES
Containing the Virus

"The name of this game is that you have to overreact."
Dr. James Young, Toronto's commissioner of public safety

Overreaction as a Policy Guideline

The battle against SARS can be said to be taking place on two fronts: on one hand, doctors, scientists and researchers worked frantically to treat infected patients and analyse the disease; on the other, governments officials formulated and implemented emergency policies on-the-fly to control the outbreak. Governments hope that containment measures would stop or at least slow down the outbreak, stalling for time so that researchers can develop a cure for the illness.

The above quote from Dr. James Young perhaps best epitomises the attitudes of government and health officials in dealing with SARS. As the rate of infection is alarmingly high, the authorities in every country are adopting strict precautionary measures, sometimes even seemingly excessive ones, to combat the disease.

Identify, Isolate and Contain

The general strategy that governments have adopted is to identify, to isolate and to contain.

One of the top priorities of governments is to identify all cases of infection and suspected cases, and then isolate them so as to prevent them from spreading the

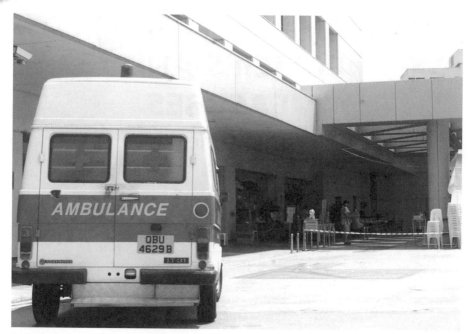

SARS Ambulance *The health authority in Singapore has specially set aside 32 ambulances for the transportation of SARS patients and suspected cases. A person who suspects that he may have contracted the disease can call for an ambulance instead of going to the hospital using public transport.*

illness to the rest of the population. The recent activities of infected patients were traced, so as to identify the people who had come into close contact with them. In several countries, such as Singapore, Hong Kong, Canada, and the US, the people who had came into close contact with infected cases were quarantined or monitored closely.

Infected patients and suspected cases were moved to specific hospitals, with exclusive teams of medical staff to tend to them. All medical staff took preventive measures such as wearing protective gear and their health was closely monitored for symptoms of infection. In addition, these hospitals, or specific wards within these hospitals, were made out-of-bounds to non-SARS related patients or staff. Strict restrictions were also implemented on visitors.

As it has been established that the disease was spread globally by air travel, many airlines and airports have implemented screening procedures. Air crew were instructed to look out for SARS symptoms among passengers, and to single them out for medical examination. Plane loads of passengers were also quarantined whenever an infected case was detected on board. Airports also adopt proactive measures like distributing flyers to passengers to inform them about the disease,

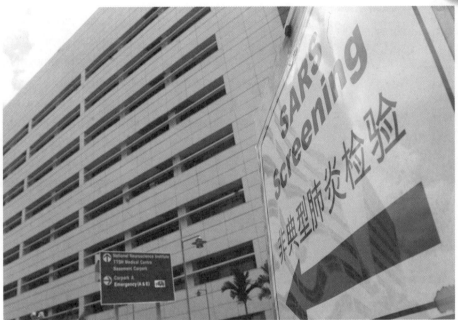

SARS Centre *In order to contain the disease, many countries have centralised all SARS patients in one or two hospitals. The above picture shows Tan Tock Seng Hospital in Singapore, which houses most of the SARS patients and functions as a screening centre as well.*

and stationing medical teams who are trained to handle suspected cases near passenger arrival halls.

Schools are places where large numbers of children congregate, and hence, are potential centres for mass infection. There was considerable parental concern about the risk of sending their children to school in SARS striken Hong Kong and Singapore. Hence, the respective governments have taken a drastic but prudent step of closing the public schools until the SARS outbreak is controlled. This was done for two reasons: to allay the fears of the parents; and to minimise the risk of further outbreak.

Similarly, the work place could also become centres of infection, especially in production

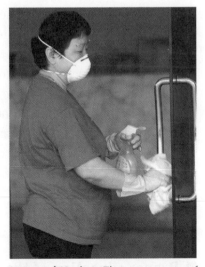

Increased Hygiene *The management of many workplaces as well as government ministries have stepped up their level of hygiene. Here, a janitor is shown disinfecting and cleaning the entrance of an office building.*

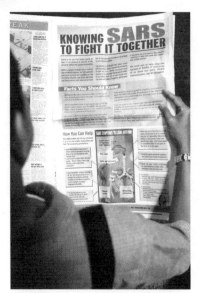

factories where workers are in close proximity with one another. Already, some companies have suspended their operations when their employees were found to be infected with SARS.

The level of public and personal hygiene has also been raised. Governments took extra care to clean and disinfect public areas such as train stations and public buses. Taxi companies urged their drivers to clean and air their vehicles thoroughly after every shift. Individuals became more conscious about washing their hands with soap regularly and refrained from excessive rubbing of their faces.

Raising Public Awareness Critical information on SARS must be made availble to the public so that individuals can take personal preventive measures.

Raising Awareness and Public Education

Governments have also launched intensive public education and awareness campaigns via the media such as newspapers, television and radio stations. Health ministries implemented measures to ensure that general practitioners and health workers were familiar with the procedures of handling SARS cases and to take precautionary measures in order to make sure that they are well-protected. The public was informed of the symptoms of SARS and to seek treatment at appropriate designated treatment centres. Organisations such as offices and schools disseminated critical information about the disease to their employees and students.

Proper education of the public on the disease can certainly serve to allay fear, squelch fallacious rumours and prevent public panic, and help foster better public understanding of the disease.

Proper education of the public on the disease can certainly serve to allay fear, squelch fallacious rumours and prevent public panic, and help foster better public understanding of the disease.

Governmental Transparency and Decisiveness

An issue that became salient due to the outbreak of SARS is governmental transparency and the authority's ability to act decisively when faced with a crisis.

Some authorities prefer to handle the situation with partial or complete secrecy, divulging little information to the public. This was done mainly for political reasons, as officials fear that a free flow of information may set off unwarranted rumours and result in public panic and consequently, social unrest. Of course, the potential damage of an epidemic to the tourist industry and prestige of the country are factored in as well.

China, the suspected place of origin of the SARS virus, has been most widely criticised for its lack of transparency in dealing with the SARS outbreak. The government gave scant information about the situation in the country and muzzled its state-controlled media. However, after international criticism mounted, the country finally relented and released statistics on the situation within its borders. It also sought the help of the WHO in dealing with the problem. Commenting on China, the director-general of WHO, Gro Harlem Brundtland, said that the Chinese should have asked for international help earlier before the deadly disease spread worldwide. The media has also chastised China for compromising the public health of both its own citizens and the international community by holding back critical information.

To a lesser extent, the authorities of Hong Kong was also accused of foot-dragging. Hong Kong was alleged to have underestimated the danger of the disease, and hence, acted too slowly. However, when the seriousness of the outbreak was realised, the government took quick and decisive actions.

Elsewhere, governments in other countries such as Singapore, Canada and the US adopted an open and transparent attitude in dealing with the health crisis. There were regular public updates as well as a relatively free flow of information from the authorities.

It is hoped that such an approach would raise public awareness and help curb the SARS outbreak more effectively. An open approach also allows better cooperation between the government and the public, as well as better coordination between different countries hit by the same disease.

Keys to Success: Coordination and Cooperation

In spite of all the institutional isolation, preventive and containment measures that governments have undertaken, it has to be understood that these "rings of defence" for combating the disease, as the Singapore authorities termed them, cannot be assumed to be foolproof. All it takes is just one case to slip through the dragnet, and a whole chain of infections could be set off in a matter of days.

However, the effectiveness of governmental preventive measures can be maximised if there is proper coordination, cooperation and implementation.

At the local level, it would take the combined effort of a determined government and a cooperative public to control the outbreak. Vigilance and pro-activeness is of utmost importance for both parties. At the international level, governments from different countries have to increase surveillance on travellers and share information as well as their own experiences with one another. It is only through a well-executed domestic effort, coupled with a well-coordinated international effort, that SARS can be brought under control.

This rest of this chapter gives a summary of the actions undertaken by health organisations and governments in different countries to combat SARS, and the policies that they have implemented to isolate infected patients and contain the virus.

Australia

- Commonwealth Department of Health and Ageing (CMO) coordinates with the WHO.
- Monitors and discloses all SARS cases.
- Warns and educates public about SARS and its symptoms.
- Intensified disease surveillance capacity by providing information on SARS to hospitals, health workers and general practitioners.

It is only through a well-executed domestic effort, coupled with a well-coordinated international effort, that SARS can be brought under control.

- Advises public against making trips to Hong Kong, Vietnam and China.
- Border and airline/airport staff briefed on infection control measures.

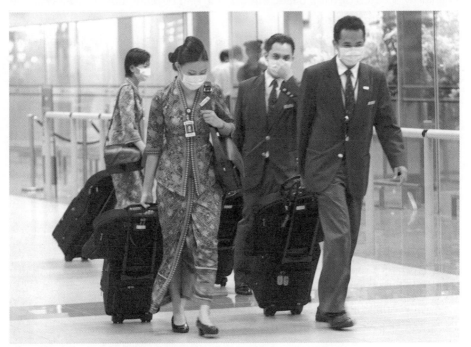

Protected *Air crew operating in affected countries wear face masks to protect themselves.*

Canada

- Coordinates with the WHO.
- Monitors and discloses all SARS cases.
- Warns and educates public about SARS and its symptoms.
- Intensified disease surveillance capacity by providing information on SARS to hospitals, health workers and General Practitioners.
- Advises public against making trips to Hong Kong, Vietnam and China.
- Access to Scarborough Grace Hospital in Toronto, where several cases were discovered, was restricted.
- Home quarantine imposed on those who have come into close contact with people diagnosed with SARS.
- Provincial and local health officials step up surveillance for new cases, especially at airports.

China

- Initially accused of withholding information and covering up the severity of the outbreak within its borders.
- Started to cooperate with the WHO after pressure from the international community.
- Provides periodic updates on SARS cases.
- Repeatedly stated that the disease was "under control".
- Efforts and precautionary measures by government still unclear.

Hong Kong

- Government initially criticised for lack of decisive action.
- Department of Health and government coordinate with the WHO.
- Monitors and discloses all SARS cases.
- Warns and educates public about SARS and its symptoms.
- Intensified disease surveillance capacity by providing information on SARS to hospitals, health workers and General Practitioners.
- Advises public against making trips to Hong Kong, Vietnam and China
- Closed all its public schools.
- Home quarantines imposed on those who have come into close contact with people diagnosed with SARS.

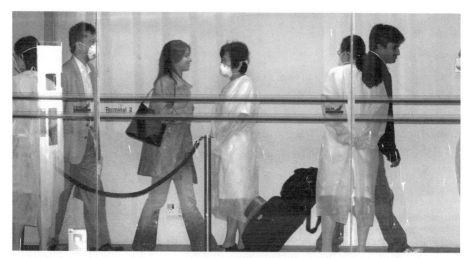

Airport Screening *Passengers arriving in Singapore Changi Airport are screened for symptoms of SARS.*
(Source: Lianhe Zaobao)

- The residents of an apartment where about 200 infected cases were found were quarantined in countryside vacation camps.
- Hewlett Packard shut down its 5-storey office when 1 worker went down with SARS.

Singapore

- Adopts a very transparent and proactive approach in tackling the problem.
- Coordinates with the WHO.
- Monitors and discloses all SARS cases.
- Warns and educates public about SARS and its symptoms.
- Intensified disease surveillance capacity by providing information on SARS to hospitals, health workers and General Practitioners.
- Advises public against making trips to Hong Kong, Vietnam and China
- All patients with SARS treated in isolation rooms in Tan Tock Seng Hospital.
- All medical staff treating SARS patients to don protective garments including masks, gloves and gowns. Doctors will even put on germ warfare suits if required.
- For all incoming flights from affected areas as identified by the WHO, nurses who are on standby will check on passengers who appear unwell. Those with fever will be sent to Tan Tock Seng Hospital for further assessment.
- A fleet of ambulances specially set aside for the transportation of SARS patients to hospitals.

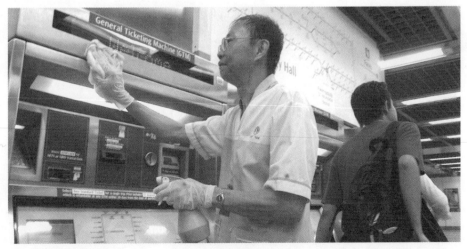

Stepping Up Cleanliness *Singapore and Hong Kong have stepped up on the level of hygiene at public places. Here, a cleaner is shown cleaning a subway station.*

- All airlines operating at Changi Airport required to screen their passengers by asking them the three questions recommended by the World Health Organisation (WHO) before allowing them to board the flight to Singapore.
- All public schools (From Primary Schools up to Junior Colleges) and government-run pre-schools suspended for a period of time.
- Home quarantine imposed on those who have come into close contact with people diagnosed with SARS.
- Ministry of Manpower advises employers to be "flexible" in handling employees who are quarantined.
- Ministerial task force formed to tackle the problem.
- Motorola suspended an entire shift from its factory when one of its workers went down with SARS.

Taiwan

- Coordinates with the WHO.
- Monitors and discloses all SARS cases.
- Warns and educates public about SARS and its symptoms.
- Intensified disease surveillance capacity by providing information on SARS to hospitals, health workers and General Practitioners.
- Advises public against making trips to Hong Kong, Vietnam and China.
- Restricted boat movement from mainland China.
- If suspected cases are found on incoming flights, the passengers and crew would be quarantined for 5 days.

United States

- Centre for Disease Control and Prevention (CDC) coordinates with WHO.
- Monitors and discloses all SARS cases.
- Warns and educates public about SARS and its symptoms.
- Intensified disease surveillance capacity by providing information on SARS to hospitals, health workers and General Practitioners.
- Advises public against making trips to Hong Kong, Vietnam, China and Singapore.
- Added SARS to the list of quarantinable communicable diseases under the Public Health Service Act.
- Non-essential travel by US officials to severely affected countries curtailed.

Vietnam

- Coordinates with the WHO.
- Monitors and discloses all SARS cases.
- Warns and educates public about SARS and it symptoms.
- Intensified disease surveillance capacity by providing information on SARS to hospitals, health workers and General Practitioners.

atbreak of SARS recently
ceed to the upper floors without any
the Management. Please wait for the
atte you at the Reception.
e caused is regre

Chapter 6

KEEPING SARS AT BAY

A Comprehensive List of Preventive Measures for Individuals and Organisations

Contents

Clinics

Residential Care Homes for the Elderly and People with Disabilities

Preventive Measures for Healthcare Professionals

Visiting Patients with Pneumonia

Preventive Measures for Conveyance Crew Members

Caring for Sick Family Members with Respiratory Illness

For Travellers

For Airlines

To All Licensees of Food Premises

To All Licensees of Non-Food Premises

Organisers of Environmental Activities

To All Hotel/Guesthouse/Holiday Flat/Holiday Camp Licensees

Guidelines for Cleansing of Private Housing Estates/Residential and Commercial Buildings
    Places Requiring Special Attention
    Places with Relatively Fewer People Gathering
    Cleansing Procedures
    General Cleansing Equipment
    Points to Note for Cleansing Staff

For the Trade and Industry Sector
    Organisational Level
    Personal Level
    Working Environment

Use of Herbal Medicines
    Preventing SARS with Traditional Chinese Medicines
    Two Prescriptions Recommended by Chinese Physicians

Acknowledgements

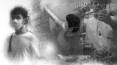

Introduction

This section provides readers with a brief background on SARS as well as comprehensive preventive guidelines, both on an individual basis and the context of various different organisations.

It is hoped that by highlighting the preventive measures, individuals and organisations can co-operate in helping to curb the virus spread.

Finally, the short section on herbal medicines is a brief collection of the recommendations made by several practising Chinese physicians in the region.

Background

Q. What is Pneumonia?

A. **Pneumonia** refers to an inflammation or infection of the lungs, which results in abnormal function. Pneumonia can be classified into typical and atypical cases.

Typical Pneumonia is usually caused by bacteria such as *Streptococcus pneumoniae*. Symptoms include sudden onset of fever, chest pain, cough and purulent sputum.

Atypical Pneumonia is usually caused by influenza virus, mycoplasma, chlamydia, adenovirus and other microbes. Common symptoms include fever, chills, cough, headache and general malaise.

Q. How contagious is SARS?

A. Based on currently available evidence, close contact with an infected person poses the highest risk of the infective agent to spread from one person to another. To date, the majority of cases have occurred in hospital workers who have cared for SARS patients and the close family members of these patients. However, the amount of the infective agent needed to cause an infection has not yet been determined.

Q.   What does WHO recommend?

A.   WHO recommends that global surveillance continues and that suspected cases are reported to national health authorities. WHO urges national health authorities to remain on the alert for suspected cases and to follow recommended protective measures. SARS patients should be isolated and cared for using barrier-nursing techniques and provided with symptomatic treatment.

Q.   Should we be worried?

A.   This illness can be severe and, due to global travel, has spread to several countries in a relatively short period of time. However, SARS is not highly contagious when protective measures are used, and the percentage of cases that have been fatal is low.

Individual Preventive Measures

As a precautionary measure, members of the public are advised to take precautionary measures to prevent respiratory tract infections:

- Build up good body immunity. This means taking a proper diet, having regular exercise and adequate rest, reducing stress and avoiding smoking;

- Maintain good personal hygiene, and wash hands after sneezing, coughing or cleaning the nose;

- Avoid touching the eyes, nose and mouth. If necessary, wash hands before touching them;

- Do not share towels;

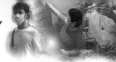

- Use serving utensils at meal times;

- Maintain good ventilation:
    - Keep air-conditioners well maintained. Wash filters frequently.
    - Open windows to improve ventilation.

- Avoid visiting crowded places with poor ventilation;

- Consult doctor promptly if not feeling well.
    - Consult a doctor promptly if there are symptoms of respiratory illness.
    - Sick children should not be taken to school or childcare centres.
    - People with respiratory tract infections should wear masks to prevent the spread of infection.
    - Carers should wear masks to reduce the chance of infection.

Wearing a Facemask

Wearing facemask properly offers satisfactory protection against respiratory tract infections. People with respiratory symptoms and those who have close contact with confirmed cases of atypical pneumonia should wear a facemask to reduce the chance of spread of infection. Their carers and those visiting sick people in hospitals should also wear a facemask. The general public may wear a facemask for self-protection.

Points to note:

1. Wash hands before wearing a facemask.

2. Follow the instructions on the package carefully, if available.

3. In general, when wearing a surgical facemask, the following should be noted:
    - The facemask should fit snugly over the face.
    - The coloured side of the facemask should face outside.
    - Tie all the strings that keep the facemask in place or fix the rubber bands of the facemask round the ears properly.
    - The facemask should fully cover the nose, mouth as well as the chin.
    - The metallic wire part of the facemask should be fixed securely over the bridge of the nose to prevent leakage.

   – Under general circumstances, the surgical mask should be changed daily.

4. Put the facemask in a plastic bag and tie the bag properly before disposing it off in a rubbish bin.

5. Replace the facemask immediately if it is damaged or soiled.

Wearing a facemask is just one of the ways to prevent respiratory tract infections. The most important thing a person should do is to observe good personal hygiene. For example, wash hands frequently with liquid soap, especially after sneezing, coughing or cleaning the nose.

Preventive Measures for Schools

(i) Pre-schools, Schools, Childcare Centres and Other Institutional Settings

   Communicable diseases (or infectious diseases) can spread among children and those who take care of them by close contact. Staff of childcare centres and schools, therefore, play an important role in the prevention, early detection and management of communicable diseases in children.

PERSONAL HYGIENE

- Cleanse used toys and furniture properly;

- Keep hands clean and wash hands properly;

- Cover nose and mouth when sneezing or coughing;

- Wash hands when they are dirtied by respiratory secretions, e.g. after sneezing;

- Use liquid soap for hand washing and disposable towel for drying hands;

- Do not share towels.

(a) Staffs at schools have to keep hands clean and fingernails trimmed.

(b) Staff should wash their hands.

   – before preparing or serving food.
   – after diapering a child or wiping his/her nose.

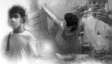

    – after cleaning up excreta or vomitus.

    – after using the toilet.

(c) Staff should make sure that children's hands are washed.

    – before eating or drinking.

    – after visiting the toilet.

    – after playing with toys or animals/pets.

    – when hands are dirtied by respiratory secretions, e.g. after sneezing.

(d) Wash hands properly.

    – Wet hands under running water.

    – Apply liquid soap and rub hands together to make a soapy lather.

    – Away from the running water, rub the front and back of hands. Massage all the fingertips properly including the thumb, the web of the fingers, around and under the nails. Do this for at least 10 seconds.

    – Rinse hands thoroughly under running water.

    – Dry hands thoroughly with a clean cotton towel, a paper towel, or a hand dryer.

    – The cleaned hands should not touch the water tap directly again. The tap may be turned off:

        • By using the towel wrapping the faucet; or

        • After splashing water to clean the faucet; or

        • By the staff.

    – Towels should never be shared. Each used towel should be properly disposed off.

    – Individuals who prefer to use their own cotton towel should make sure that their towel is not shared with others. It is preferable to have more than one towel for each day's use. The towels should be washed at least once daily.

• Cover mouth and nose with handkerchiefs while sneezing and coughing.

• Keep hairs clean and tidy.

• Wear gloves when handling wounds, nose bleeding and soiled articles; wash hands afterwards.

- Keep personal items like towels separate from one another.

- Never share towels, handkerchiefs, toothbrushes, or eating utensils or other personal items.

- Avoid picking the nose and rubbing the eyes.

(ii) Guidelines on the Prevention of the Spreading of Atypical Pneumonia in Schools

A.   **Civic Education**
      Prevent the Spreading of Atypical Pneumonia: Schools as a Start

A.1   Explain to staff and students the importance of hygiene in preventing infection, especially in preventing the infection of atypical pneumonia. State the serious consequences of the spreading of atypical pneumonia in the region. Emphasise that everyone in the community has the responsibility to prevent the spreading of atypical pneumonia. Encourage staff and students to seek medical advice immediately, and notify the school and the Department of Health, in case of any suspected infection of atypical pneumonia involving themselves or their families.

A.2   Include relevant topics on the prevention of infectious disease /atypical pneumonia in the learning activities. Adopt diverse learning modes to enhance the students' awareness and concern. Staff and students should be reminded to put their knowledge into practice and to heed personal hygiene in order to avoid infection. They should also convey the message to relatives and friends.

A.3   Disseminate the message to parents through seminars or newsletters, and distribute to them leaflets or relevant materials published by the Education and Manpower Bureau (EMB) or other organisations concerned. The students and their parents should be provided with such information as the hotline numbers and web sites of the appropriate government authorities.

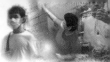

B. Precautionary Measures

B.1 Schools should formulate precautionary and contingency measures on the basis of the content in the circular memoranda issued to schools. Staff, students and parents should be informed of these measures, and symptoms of atypical pneumonia should be described in particular. It should be highlighted that children with fever should not go to school and must consult their doctors immediately.

B.2 Students should be reminded to be aware of their own or their classmates' physical condition during assembly or class periods. If they are unwell, they should inform their teachers and classmates immediately. Students should also be reminded not to eat from the same lunch box or drink from the same cup to avoid infection.

B.3 Maintain good cleanliness and ventilation in the school hall and classrooms. Windows should be kept open. Air filters should be cleansed frequently if air-conditioners are used. Objects and equipment frequently touched by students, such as computer keyboards, should be wiped regularly in diluted household bleach. Toys of pupils should be soaked regularly using diluted household bleach. If a school bus is used to carry pupils to the school, good cleanliness and sanitation of the vehicle compartment should be ensured as well.

B.4 Liquid soap should be provided in the toilets. Public towels should not be used. Notice should be posted to require staff and students to use liquid soap for hand washing to avoid infection.

B.5 In organising internal or external group activities, good ventilation of the venue should be taken into account. Crowds should be avoided. Students who are unwell should be persuaded to avoid participating in school activities.

B.6 Keep an up-to-date sick leave record of students and staff and obtain their prior consent for the release of personal data, such as names and telephone numbers to the DH for investigation and follow-up action.

B.7 If a student or staff member is unwell (including school bus driver and school bus assistant), (s)he should be sent to an isolated and quiet place for rest. Their family members should be contacted to take them home. In the case of a student, (s)he should be sent home with a note suggesting medical attention. If the student is with a fever or seriously ill, (s)he should be sent to the Accident and Emergency Department of a nearby hospital if parents/guardians cannot be contacted.

B.8 Caretakers of staff and students who are unwell should put on masks to avoid infection.

B.9 In case of an unusual increase in absenteeism or where a large number of absentees with symptoms similar to atypical pneumonia are noted, e.g. fever, cough, headache, body pain and lack of energy, the relevant government authorities should be notified immediately.

Preventive Measures for Public Transport Operators

- Public transport operators are advised to take the following precautionary measures for vehicles to prevent respiratory infections:
  - Maintain good personal hygiene. Cover the nose and mouth when sneezing or coughing.
  - Wash hands after sneezing, coughing or cleaning the nose.
  - Avoid touching the eyes, nose and mouth. If necessary, wash hands before touching them.
  - Consult the doctor promptly and take sick leave if you develop symptoms of respiratory tract infection.

- Maintaining good ventilation on vehicles:
  - Open the windows whenever possible to ensure good ventilation.
  - For closed vehicle compartments, clean the air-conditioning system frequently to maintain good functioning.

- Keeping vehicle compartments clean:
  - Wash/wipe vehicle compartments with diluted domestic bleach (mixing 1 part of bleach with 99 parts of water) regularly.
  - Make tissue paper available for passengers' use when necessary.
  - Make vomit bags available for passengers' use.
  - If vehicle compartments are contaminated with vomitus, wash/wipe with

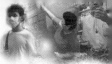

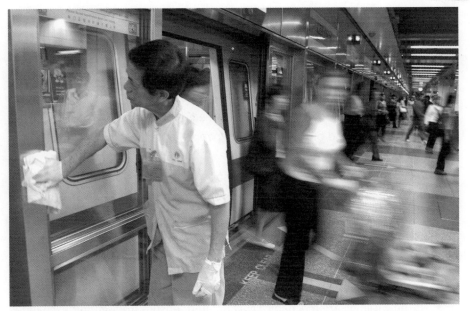

Cleaning the Train Station *The SMRT (Singapore Mass Rapid Transit) has stepped up the cleanliness of its subway stations.*

diluted domestic bleach (mixing 1 part of bleach with 49 parts of water) immediately.

- Please advise passengers as follows:
  - Observe personal hygiene. Cover the nose and mouth with handkerchief or tissue paper when sneezing or coughing.
  - Dispose off used tissue paper properly.
  - Use a vomit bag to hold vomitus and dispose off it properly.
  - Consult the doctor promptly if they develop symptoms of respiratory tract infection.

Preventive Measures When Using Public Transport

As a precautionary measure, members of the public are advised to take the following measures to prevent respiratory tract infections:

- Build up good body immunity by having a proper diet, regular exercise and adequate rest, reducing stress and avoiding smoking.
- Maintain good personal hygiene, and wash hands after sneezing, coughing or cleaning the nose.

- Avoid touching the eyes, nose and mouth. If necessary, wash hands before touching them.
- Maintain good ventilation.
- Avoid visiting crowded places with poor ventilation.
- Consult their doctor promptly if they develop respiratory symptoms.
- Patients with respiratory symptoms are advised to wear mask to reduce the chance of spread of the infection to people around them.

As millions of people use the public transport system everyday, it is particularly important that public transport companies and operators ensure good ventilation and cleanliness in the vehicle compartment and station facilities. Specific advice on the prevention of diseases is highlighted below:

- Plenty of fresh air should be introduced into the vehicle compartment and station facilities;
- If the facilities are mechanically ventilated, ensure frequent air exchanges and proper maintenance and cleansing of the system;
- Cleanse and disinfect furniture and vehicle compartment regularly (at least once a day), using diluted household bleach (i.e. adding 1 part of household bleach to 99 parts of water), rinse with water and then mop dry.

Preventive Measures in Public Places

Members of the public are advised to avoid crowded public places in order to prevent the spread of respiratory tract infections.

Visiting Public Places

When visiting crowded places such as cinemas and restaurants, the following precautionary measures should be taken:

- Maintain good personal hygiene. Cover nose and mouth when sneezing or coughing.
- Dispose off used tissue paper properly.
- Keep hands clean. Wash hands when they are dirtied by respiratory secretions e.g. after sneezing.

- Avoid touching the eyes, nose and mouth. If necessary, wash hands before touching them.
- Do not share towels.
- Use serving utensils at meal times.
- Consult your doctor promptly if you develop respiratory symptoms, and follow instructions given by your doctor including the use of drugs as prescribed and adequate rest as appropriate.
- Patients should put on masks to reduce the chance of spread of infection.

Working in Public Places

Workers in public places should take the following precautionary measures to reduce the chance of spread of infection:

- Maintain good personal hygiene. Cover nose and mouth when sneezing or coughing.
- Wash hands after sneezing, coughing or cleaning the nose.
- Avoid touching the eyes, nose and mouth. If necessary, wash hands before touching them.
- Consult your doctor promptly and take sick leave if you develop respiratory symptoms.
- Allow plenty of fresh air into the indoor environment.
- If the facilities are mechanically ventilated, ensure frequent air exchanges and proper maintenance and cleansing of the system.
- Ensure that toilet flushing apparatus is functioning properly.
- Provide toilets with liquid soap and disposable tissue towels or hand dryers.
- Cleanse and disinfect the facilities (including furniture and toilet facilities) regularly (at least once a day), using diluted household bleach (i.e. adding 1 part of household bleach to 99 parts of water), rinse with water and then mop dry.
- If the facilities are contaminated with vomitus, wash/wipe with diluted domestic bleach (mixing 1 part of bleach with 49 parts of water) immediately.

Preventive Measures for Property Services Companies

Health Advice to All Housing Residents

Advice should be given through newsletters and notices to urge public housing residents to take the following precautionary measures:

- Build up good body immunity by having a balanced diet, regular exercise and adequate rest, reducing stress and avoiding smoking.
- Maintain good personal hygiene. Cover the nose and mouth when sneezing or coughing.
- Wash hands before touching eyes, mouth and nose.
- Keep hands clean and wash hands properly. Use liquid soap for hand washing and disposable towel for drying hands.
- Wash hands if dirtied by respiratory secretions (e.g. after sneezing).
- Do not share towels.
- Keep the home environment clean, and cleanse furniture properly.
- Maintain good indoor ventilation.
- Avoid visiting crowded places with poor ventilation.
- Put on masks and consult the doctor promptly if symptoms like fever, cough, etc. developed.

Maintaining Good Ventilation in Public Places

- Open the windows in public places whenever possible to ensure good ventilation.
- Cleanse air-conditioning systems such as air-conditioners and exhaust fans frequently to maintain their good functioning.
- For central air-conditioning systems, ensure frequent air exchanges and proper maintenance and cleansing of the systems.

Keeping Lift Cars and Escalators in Public Housing Estates Clean

- Wipe lift cars and escalators, particularly call buttons and handrails, regularly with 1:99 diluted household bleach (i.e. adding 1 part of bleach to 99 parts of water), not less than twice daily.

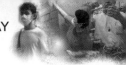

- If lift cars and escalators are contaminated with vomitus, wash/wipe with 1:49 diluted household bleach (i.e. adding 1 part of bleach to 49 parts of water) immediately.
- Cleanse the exhaust fans at the ceiling of the lift cars to maintain their good functioning.

Cleaning Corridors and Public Areas in Estates

- By holding activities under Operation Fire Exit Staircase, take prompt actions in one week to clean the corridors and public areas in estates with 1:99 diluted household bleach (i.e. adding 1 part of bleach to 99 parts of water), rinse with water and then mop them dry.
- Afterwards, carry out cleansing exercises once every two weeks with 1:99 diluted household bleach.

Cleaning Shopping Centres, Markets and Car Parks

- Take prompt actions in three days to clean the public areas of shopping centres, markets and car parks in estates thoroughly with 1:99 diluted household bleach (i.e. adding 1 part of bleach to 99 parts of water), rinse with water and then mop them dry.
- Afterwards, carry out cleansing exercises daily with 1:99 diluted household bleach (i.e. adding 1 part of bleach to 99 parts of water), rinse with water and then mop them dry.

Other Common Facilities that Should be Attended To

- Ensure that the toilet flushing apparatus is functioning properly.
- Provide toilets with liquid soap and disposable tissue towels or hand dryers.
- Ensure proper cleansing and maintenance of the toilet exhaust system.
- Cleanse and disinfect recreational facilities and benches in estates regularly with 1:99 diluted household bleach (i.e. adding 1 part of bleach to 99 parts of water), rinse with water and then mop them dry.
- Equipment in estate offices should be wiped and cleaned twice a day with 1:99 diluted household bleach (i.e. adding 1 part of bleach to 99 parts of water).

Clinics

- All clinic staff should enforce strict infection control measures appropriate for their particular setting, especially observance of good personal hygiene.

- If staff fall sick, they should report to their seniors and take sick leave as appropriate.

- Where considered necessary, for example, treating or nursing a patient with respiratory symptoms, staff may wear masks.

- The Department of Health will continue to monitor the situation of the pneumonia cases and issue advice accordingly.

- Patients with respiratory symptoms are advised to wear mask to reduce the chance of spread of the infection.

Residential Care Homes for the Elderly and People with Disabilities

For diseases spread by airborne of direct contact transmission

- Maintain good indoor ventilation.
- Keep hands clean and wash hands properly.
- Cleanse used furniture properly.
- Dispose off used tissue paper properly, cover nose and mouth when sneezing or coughing.
- Wash hands when they are dirtied by respiratory secretions e.g. after sneezing.
- Prevent head lice by keeping hair clean.
- Prevent scabies by regular bathing.
- Keep personal cleanliness.
- Wash hands properly after handling each resident, e.g. after applying medication or changing diaper.
- Wash linen of residents infected with scabies separately.
- Do not share towels.

Preventive Measures for Healthcare Professionals

- Masking
  - All staff should wear a surgical mask;
  - Patients should be asked to wear a mask if they have respiratory symptoms.
- Hand Washing with Liquid Soap
  - Before and after patient contact;
  - After removing gloves.
- Wear Gloves
  - For all direct patient contacts;
  - Change gloves between patients and wash hands.
- Wear Gown
  - During procedures likely to generate splashes or sprays of blood and body fluid, secretion or excretions.
- Eye Protection
  - For aerosol/splash generating procedures.
- Avoidance of Aerosols
  - Do not use nebulisers in patients with symptoms compatible with SARS.
- Environmental Disinfection
  - Clean surfaces daily with a disinfectant, e.g. 1:49 diluted household bleach, sodium hypochlorite 1000 ppm or 70% alcohol for metallic surfaces.
- Disease Detection
  - Seek medical attention promptly if symptoms compatible with SARS (e.g. fever, chills, myalgia, shortness of breath and difficulty in breathing).

Visiting Patients with Pneumonia

- Visitors to warded patients are advised to take due precautions in infection control, e.g. wearing facemask and gowns and to wash hands thoroughly afterwards before coming into contact with other people.

Preventive Measures for Conveyance Crew Members

Crew members of conveyances (aircraft, vessel, etc.) who notice a passenger seriously ill with a respiratory illness should:

- Keep the ill passenger away from other passengers as much as possible.
- Provide a surgical mask, if available, for the ill passenger to wear to reduce the number of droplets coughed into the air.
- Alternatively, ask the passengers to cover their mouth and nose with tissues provided when coughing.
- Remember to wash hands with soap and water after contact with the ill passenger.

Crew members should be aware of symptoms of Severe Acute Respiratory Syndrome, i.e. fever (>38°C) **AND** cough, shortness of breath, or breathing difficulty. If you become ill and you are concerned about Severe Acute Respiratory Syndrome, see your family doctor and inform about your possible exposure.

The captain is reminded to report the illness to the port health authority of the destination. Port health officials will arrange for appropriate medical assistance on arrival of the conveyance.

Caring for Sick Family Members with Respiratory Illness

- Patients should consult a doctor if they are unwell.

- They should follow instructions given by the doctor including the use of drugs as prescribed and taking adequate rest as appropriate.

- Adhere to good personal hygiene practices.

- Ensure adequate ventilation.

- Patients should put on masks to reduce the chances of spread of infection to carers.

- Carers may also put on masks to reduce the chances of acquiring infection through the airways.

For Travellers

All out-bound and in-bound travellers should be aware of the main symptoms and signs of Severe Acute Respiratory Syndrome which include:

- High fever (>38°C) **AND**
- One or more respiratory symptoms including cough, shortness of breath, difficulty breathing **AND**
- Close contact* with a person who has been diagnosed with Severe Acute Respiratory Syndrome, OR have a recent history of travel to areas reporting cases of Severe Acute Respiratory Syndrome.

In addition to fever and respiratory symptoms, Severe Acute Respiratory Syndrome may be associated with other symptoms including headache, muscular stiffness, loss of appetite, malaise, confusion, rash, and diarrhoea.

In the unlikely event of a traveller experiencing this combination of symptoms they should seek medical attention and ensure that information about their recent travel is passed on to the health care staff. Any traveller who develops these symptoms is advised not to undertake further travel until they have recovered.

Any sick passenger identified during flight would on arrival be referred to the airport health authorities. Other fellow passengers and crew on the aircraft should provide all contact details for the subsequent 14 days to the airport health authorities.

It is prudent for tourists to adopt the following precautionary measures to prevent atypical pneumonia, including Severe Acute Respiratory Syndrome:

- Build up good body immunity by having a proper diet, regular exercise and adequate rest, reducing stress and avoiding smoking.
- Maintain good personal hygiene, and wash hands after sneezing, coughing or cleaning the nose.
- Avoid touching the eyes, nose and mouth. If necessary, wash hands before touching them.
- Maintain good ventilation.
- Avoid visiting crowded places with poor ventilation.
- Do not share towels or eating utensils.
- Consult a doctor promptly if you develop respiratory symptoms.

---

* Close contact means having cared for, having lived with, or having had direct contact with respiratory secretions and body fluids of a person with Severe Acute Respiratory Syndrome.

The World Health Organisation recommends, on 2 April 2003, that persons travelling to Hong Kong and Guangdong Province of China consider postponing non-essential travel. This temporary recommendation does not apply to passengers directly transiting through international airports within these areas.

For Airlines

Should a passenger or crew member who meets the criteria above travel on a flight, the aircraft should alert the destination airport. On arrival the sick passenger should be referred to airport health authorities for assessment and management. The aircraft passengers and crew should be informed of the person's status as a suspect case of Severe Acute Respiratory Syndrome. The passengers and crew should provide all contact details for the subsequent 14 days to the airport health authorities.

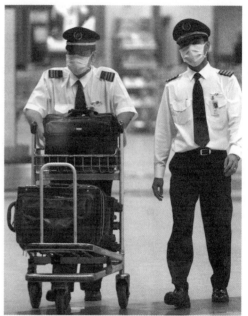
Pilots with masks

To All Licensees of Food Premises

This category includes Food Permittees, Canteen Operators and Market Store Tenants.

The licensees of the premises are urged to adopt the following measures immediately to protect the health of staff and customers:

- Step up cleaning, inspection and maintenance for all ventilating systems in the premises, including air outlets, air filters, fresh air inlets and ventilating ducts.
- Keep the ventilating systems of the premises in operation during business hours.
- In addition to providing customers with tableware for their own use, licensees of restaurants and factory canteens should also take the initiative to provide

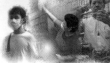

customers with additional chopsticks or spoons for the common serving of food.

- Tableware/towels provided to customers must be thoroughly washed and sterilised before re-use.
- Step up cleansing and disinfection of the walls, floors, utensils, tables, chairs and equipment on the premises.
- Any employee found suffering from respiratory tract illness should cease work immediately and consult a registered medical practitioner.
- All food, beverage and tableware must be stored and covered properly.

To All Licensees of Non-Food Premises

The licensees of the premises are urged to adopt the following measures immediately to protect the health of your staff and customers:

- Step up cleaning, inspection and maintenance for all ventilating systems in the premises, including air outlets, air filters, fresh air inlets and ventilating ducts.
- Keep the ventilating systems of the premises in operation during business hours.
- Facilities/towels provided to customers must be thoroughly washed and sterilised before re-use.
- Step up cleansing and disinfection of the walls, floors, utensils, tables, chairs and equipment on the premises.
- Any employee found suffering from respiratory tract illness should cease work immediately and consult a registered medical practitioner.

Organisers of Environmental Activities

- Maintain good personal hygiene. Cover the nose and mouth when sneezing or coughing.
- Wash hands after sneezing, coughing or cleaning the nose.
- Consult the doctor promptly if you develop symptoms of respiratory tract infection.
- Persons with symptoms of respiratory infection are advised to wear a mask to reduce the chance of spread of the infection.
- Maintain good ventilation at the venue of the event.
- Keep the venue clean, and make tissue paper and vomit bags available for use by the visitors and event participants when necessary.

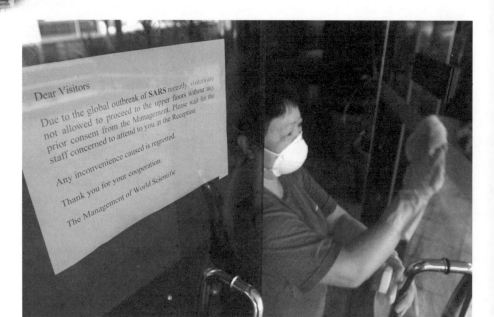

Cleaning Entrance *Special attention should be paid to doors and door knobs.*

- Please advise the visitors and event participants as follows:
  - Observe personal hygiene. Cover the nose and mouth with handkerchief or tissue paper when sneezing or coughing.
  - Dispose off used tissue paper properly.
  - Use a vomit bag to hold vomitus and dispose off it properly.
  - Consult the doctor promptly if they develop symptoms of respiratory tract infection.

To All Hotel/Guesthouse/Holiday Flat/ Holiday Camp Licensees

This includes all club certificates of compliance holders, all bedspace apartment licensees.

The licensees are urged to adopt the following measures immediately to protect the health of staff and customers:

- Step up cleaning, inspection and maintenance for all ventilating systems in the premises, including air outlets, air filters, fresh air inlets and ventilating ducts.
- Wash the pillow covers, bed sheets and blankets regularly. When customers

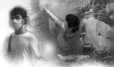

check out from the hotel/guesthouse/holiday flat/holiday camp, please wash the used pillows covers, bed sheets and blankets as soon as possible.

If you provide food and beverage to your customers, please adopt the following measures immediately:

- In addition to providing customers with tableware for their own use, you should also take the initiative to provide customers with additional chopsticks or spoons for the common serving of food.
- Tableware/towels provided to customers must be thoroughly washed and sterilised before re-use.
- Step up cleansing and disinfection of the walls, floors, utensils, tables, chairs and equipment on the premises.
- Any employee found suffering from respiratory tract illness should cease work immediately and consult a registered medical practitioner.
- All food, beverage and tableware must be stored and covered properly.

Guidelines for Cleansing of Private Housing Estates/ Residential and Commercial Buildings

(1) Places Requiring Special Attention

- Lift Car and Escalator
  - Wipe lift cars and escalators, particularly call buttons and handrails at least twice daily.
  - Cleanse the ventilating fans at the ceiling of the lift cars regularly to maintain their good functioning.
- Main Entrance Lobby
  - Wash and wipe the estate/building entrance, the door knobs/handles and the security locks and buttons thereat at least twice daily.
- Common Facility

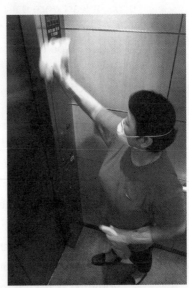

Cleaning a Lift Lifts should be cleaned regularly and thoroughly, with special attention being paid to the panel buttons.

- Wash and wipe the chairs, resting areas and other facilities used by the public in lift lobbies, corridors and public areas at least twice daily.
- Security Guard Booth and Inquiry Counter
  - Wash and wipe the security guard booths and inquiry counters at least twice daily.
- Refuse Collection Chamber
  - Dispose off daily waste and junk properly. Wash the refuse collection chambers and related facilities at least twice daily.
- Toilet
  - Wash the toilet and its facilities at least twice daily.
- Children's Playground
  - Wash and wipe the children's playground and facilities at least twice daily.

(2) Places with Relatively Fewer People Gathering

- Corridor and Public Place
  - Wash and wipe the corridors and public places (including rear staircases) at least once daily.
- Shopping Centre, Market and Car Park
  - Wash and wipe the public places of shopping centres, markets and car parks at least once daily.
- Club Facility
  - Wash and wipe the club facilities at least once daily.

(3) Cleansing Procedures

- Washing
  - Step 1

    Sweep litter before washing.
  - Step 2

    Flush with clean water.
  - Step 3

    Wash thoroughly with 1:99 (i.e. mixing 1 part of bleach with 99 parts of water) diluted household bleach. If places dirtied with filth (e.g. vomitus), 1:49 (i.e. mixing 1 part of bleach with 49 parts of water) diluted household bleach should be applied.

– Step 4

Hose down and remove excess water by mop drying or squeegee.

– Step 5

If necessary, washing should be repeated to ensure the place is thoroughly cleansed. Use high-pressure hot water cleaners as appropriate.

- Wiping
  - Step 1

    Wipe thoroughly with 1:99 (i.e. mixing 1 part with bleach with 99 parts of water) diluted household bleach. For places dirtied with filth (e.g. vomitus), 1:49 (i.e. mixing 1 part with bleach to 49 parts of water) diluted household bleach should be applied.

  - Step 2

    Wipe dry.

(4) General Cleansing Equipment

- Brush
- Mop
- Squeegee
- Bucket
- Towel
- Bleach
- Mouth mask
- Gloves
- Footwear

(5) Points to Note for Cleansing Staff

- Under normal conditions, apply 1:99 (i.e. mixing 1 part of bleach with 99 parts of water) diluted household bleach.
- For places dirtied with filth (e.g. vomitus), 1:49 (i.e. mixing 1 part with bleach to 49 parts of water) diluted household bleach should be applied.
- While at work, all staff should wear proper protective gear such as mouth mask, gloves, overall, footwear, etc.

For the Trade and Industry Sector

Organisational Level
- Consult a doctor immediately if falling sick and take leave as appropriate.
- Persons with symptoms of respiratory infection should be advised to wear a mask to reduce the chances of spread of the infection, and the persons handling those with symptoms are advised to wear a disposable surgical mask and sterile disposable gloves, and wash hands thoroughly with soap and water immediately afterwards.
- If wearing masks, ensure that it fits snugly over the nose and face area.

Personal Level
- Build up good body immunity by having a proper diet, regular exercise and adequate rest, reducing stress and avoiding smoking.
- Maintain good personal hygiene, cover nose and mouth when sneezing or coughing and wash hands after sneezing, coughing, cleaning the nose or going to toilets.
- Use serving utensils at meal times to avoid spread of the virus.
- Avoid visiting crowded places with poor ventilation.

Working Environment
- Maintain good ventilation.
- If the facilities are mechanically ventilated, ensure frequent air exchanges and proper maintenance and cleansing of the system.
- Provide toilets with liquid soap and disposable tissue towels or hand dryers.
- Ensure that toilet-flushing apparatus is functioning well.
- Cleanse and disinfect the facilities (including telephone, furniture and toilet facilities) regularly (at least once a day), using 1:99 diluted household bleach (i.e. adding 1 part of household bleach to 99 parts of water), rinse with water and then mop dry.
- If the facilities are contaminated with vomitus, disinfect immediately with 1:49 diluted household bleach (i.e. adding 1 part of household bleach to 49 parts of water), rinse with water and then mop dry.

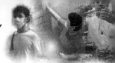

Use of Herbal Medicines

Preventing SARS with Traditional Chinese Medicine

Many Chinese subscribe to the Yin-Yang School of thought or the School of Positive and Negative Forces whose roots can be traced back to the Period of the Warring States in Chinese history (475-221 B.C). It is the interaction of yin and yang which produces all things and dissolve all things, they claim.

Yin is the negative and dark force and refers to feminine elements, while yang is the positive and bright side that is masculine. Such belief permeates Chinese life and a balance of yin and yang is thought to be essential to health. A deficiency of either principle then manifests as disease.

In the case of Severe Acute Respiratory Syndrome (SARS), while experts in Chinese medicine in different parts of the world have not arrived at a definitive way to cure the illness, Chinese medicine is perceived as capable of "clearing the heat" (or suppressing the yang that has been too much in abundance and thus upsetting the balance) and "tonifying" the lungs, as well as building up a person's immune system in this critical fight against SARS.

Chinese physicians generally regard SARS as a disease resulting from a body

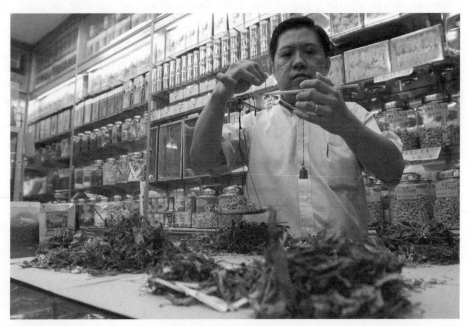

Traditional Remedy *Many people turn to Chinese herbs to strengthen their immune system. Demand for certain herbs surged dramatically, resulting in some herbs being sold out in many places.*

being exposed to external forces, which are tepid in nature. The vital energy (zheng qi, 正气) in a body fights the external forces, creating "heat" in the process and it is this "toxic heat" that attacks the respiratory system causing a person to sneeze and cough. The external forces also clog the main and collateral channels through which energy circulates, leading a person experiencing bodily aches and tiring him out.

Chinese physicians focus on methods that could "clear and purge heat", detoxicate and treat the yin deficiency, thus alleviating the medical conditions of a patient. Many types of Chinese medicines sold like hot cakes. Such Chinese medicines include isatis roots (ban lan gen, 板蓝根), wild chrysanthemum, selfheal spike (xia ku cao, 夏枯草), da qing ye 大青叶), almond, weeping forsythia (lian qiao, 连翘) and ephedra sinica (ma huang, 麻黄).

According to The Big Dictionary of Chinese Medicines (中药大词典), edited by Jiangsu New Hospital, isatis roots are consumed to "clear heat", detoxicate, "cool blood" and are used mainly to treat influenza, pneumonia, rashes and throat inflammation. They originate from Hebei, Jiangsu and Anhui in China. It is believed that when used together with apozem (jian ji, 煎剂) or with da ye qing and notopterygium roots (qiang huo, 羌活) isatis roots may help treat SARS. However, there are also cases that suggest that isatis roots may not be suitable for use by everyone as some people may develop allergies.

He Xianliang (何显亮), a Chinese physician from Hong Kong, has commented that Chinese herbs such as isatis roots and honeysuckle (jin yin hua, 金银花) could directly kill viruses and are effective in treating inflammations. They can boost immunity at the same time, but he pointed out that isatis roots may prove too "cooling" for some and continual over-consumption for days could lead to dizziness, worsen a person's health, and even affect male potency. He suggested consuming drinks with chestnut, sugarcane and others.

The following is a list of recommended list of Chinese herbs for the prevention of SARS. However, it may be advisable for one to consult opinions of Chinese physicians before consumption, and to bear in mind that the herbs are not to be consumed in large amounts.

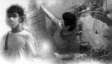

Three Prescriptions Recommended by Chinese Physicians:

Prescription I

Content	Amount
Honeysuckle (jin yin hua, 金银花)	30 g
Isatis roots (ban lan gen, 板蓝根)	10 g
Rhizoma polystichi (guan zhong, 贯众)	10 g
Almond	10 g
Ji geng (吉梗)	10 g
Ophiopogon japonicus (mai dong 麦冬)	15 g
Orange peel (chen pi, 陈皮)	6 g
Sheng gan cao (生甘草)	6 g
Hang ju hua (杭菊花)	6 g

Direction of Use

Use 300 ml of water and mix to boil till 100 g is left, consume twice a day, morning and night.

(Information provided by Zhang Wenqu, Chinese medical professor in Shenzhen)

Prescription II

Content	Amount
Betel (bing lang, 槟榔)	6 g
Pachydermia (hou pu, 厚朴)	6 g
Cao guo ren (草果仁)	3 g
Rhizoma anemarrhenae (zhi mu, 知母)	6 g
Radix paeoniae alba (bai shao, 白芍)	6 g
Huang ling (黄苓)	6 g
Liqorice (gan cao, 甘草)	3 g

Direction of Use

Use two bowls of water and mix to boil, then use a weaker flame to boil for another 5 to 10 minutes. Consume when medicine is lukewarm. After consumption, drink water every hour.

(Information provided by Dr Chen Hongneng of Singapore's ECM Chinese Medical Centre Pte Ltd)

Prescription III

Provided by Professor Xie Ming from the Beijing University of Chinese Medicine.

A. Suitable for the General Public

Content	Amount
Yin hua（银花）	9 g
Astragalus mongholicus (huang qi, 黄芪)	10–12 g
Saposhirukovia divaricata (fang feng, 防风)	6 g
Bai shu (白术)	9 g
Golden bell (liang qiao, 连翘)	9 g
Rhizoma phragmitis (lu gen, 芦根)	15–20 g
Field mint (bohe, 薄荷)	6 g
Root of balloon flower (jie gen, 桔梗)	6 g

Direction of Use

Brew using water.
Bring to boil and consume when lukewarm.

Consumption

- Consume half of dosage at a time, two times a day.
- Total dosage — 5 consecutive days.

B. Suitable for Those with a Thick Loading on the Tongue

Content	Amount
Cang shu (苍术)	9 g
Huo xiang (藿香)	9 g
Yin hua (银花)	9 g
Astragalus mongholicus (huang qi, 黄芪)	9 g
Saposhirukovia divaricata (fang feng, 防风)	6 g
Seed of job's tears (yi ren, 苡仁)	9 g
Golden bell (liang qiao, 连翘)	9 g
Rhizoma phragmitis (lu gen, 芦根)	15 g
Root of balloon flower (jie gen, 桔梗)	6 g
Toasted liquorice (zhi gan cao, 炙甘草)	5 g

Direction of Use

> Brew using water.
> Bring to boil and consume when lukewarm.

Consumption

- Consume half of dosage at a time, two times a day.
- Total dosage — 5 consecutive days.

Apart from consuming Chinese herbs, Chinese physicians advise the public to:

- avoid oily and deep fried food;
- have adequate rest;
- be aware of changes in climate;
- allow sufficient ventilation.

Professor Li Zhizhong, a Chinese physician who lectures to clinicians at the Hong Kong Baptist University pointed out on the web that diseases would not result if a person were to pay attention to the points raised above. In an interview with the press, he pointed out that the best preventive measure is to drink a lot of water.

Acknowledgements

We would like to thank the Government of the Hong Kong Special Administrative Region for granting us permission to use the contents of the displayed materials produced by the Department of Health. The brief background (Q&A) was extracted from the World Health Organisation (WHO) website.

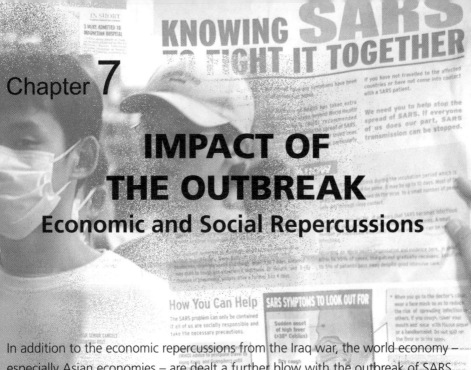

Chapter 7

IMPACT OF THE OUTBREAK
Economic and Social Repercussions

In addition to the economic repercussions from the Iraq war, the world economy – especially Asian economies – are dealt a further blow with the outbreak of SARS.

Travel

The most direct impact is the travel advisory issued by non-SARS affected countries to advise their citizens against travelling to places that are SARS-affected unless absolutely necessary. Countries such as Hong Kong, Singapore, Vietnam, Guangdong Province in China, Toronto in Canada are expected to be hardest-hit by the travel advisories. Visitors and tourist numbers to these countries are expected to decline drastically. As a consequence, Asian tourism is in a crisis.

Hotels and Airlines

Across Southeast Asia, airlines and hotels are facing massive cancellations. Travel and tourism-related businesses such as retail, restaurant and entertainment industries are most severely affected by the disease.

Singapore Airlines has announced that it will drastically cut the number of flights to various destinations. Malaysian Airlines is also cutting flights to Singapore and Hong Kong. Air Canada filed for bankruptcy citing the Iraq war and SARS. Cathay Pacific Airways is cutting flights to eight destinations including Tokyo, Manila, Taipei and Kuala Lumpur.

Travel agencies and tour groups are seeing vacation cancellations and changes in itineraries. Many hotels — already seeing a huge drop in occupancy rate for March due to the Iraq war – are experiencing worsening occupancy rate.

Government workers from some countries are banned from travelling to SARS-affected places. Many private enterprises have issued travel bans to their employees and resorted to videophones or teleconferencing to communicate with business partners and employees in other countries.

Retail and Entertainment

Apart from the reduction in business from tourists and travellers, the retail industry is also seeing a large number of people keeping away from public and crowded places in order to avoid catching the deadly flu-like disease. Places that are typically crowded on weedends – shopping centers, malls, restaurants and recreational facilities such as movie theatres and swimming pools and parks – are unusually empty. Most people are refraining from going outdoors unless necessary or to go to work. There are even stories of some people opting for self-voluntary quarantine and getting all their essential groceries through online shopping.

Across Asia, music concerts, entertainment events and business conferences are all being cancelled or postponed. This includes the World Economic Forum business meeting in Beijing, which has been postponed to September 2003 or October 2003. A major trade show to be held in Guangzhou in mid-April 2003 is also severely curtailed. US toy companies such as Mattel and Hasbro are restricting or cancelling flights to the trade show. In Switzerland, the World Jewellery & Watch Fair 2003 has banned Hong Kong exhibitors from turning up. Concerts by the rock band the Rolling Stones have been cancelled in Hong Kong, Shanghai and Beijing. Concert by Carlos Santana is also cancelled in Singapore.

Cancellation of Rolling Stones World Tour 2003

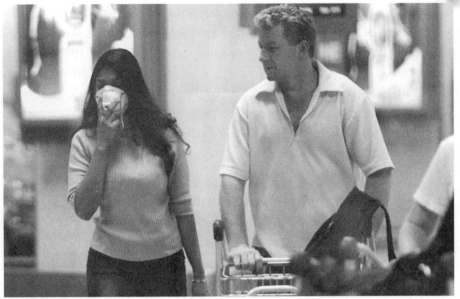

Passenger at airport way of SARS virus.

Quarantine & Shutting-Down of Schools

In addition, some governments have ordered the shutting down of schools and pre-schools as well as serving quarantine on people who are in close contact with SARS. Frenzied parents who are unable to arrange for childcare are forced to take leave from work to care for their children. All these have similar effects as a workforce strike or lock-out – a slow-down of productivity in the economy. In addition, some countries, such as Malaysia, have announced freezing the hiring of workers from SARS affected countries. The Cabinet-level Council of Labor Affairs in Taiwan has also decided to halt visas for Vietnamese workers should the situation in Vietnam worsens.

Trade & Stocks

International trade is also affected. Many American companies with trade totalling $13.4 billion with China (third largest behind Canada and Mexico) are fearing the impact on manufacturing and production. A slowdown or halt of production of goods such as apparels and video games is much dreaded.

The stocks for air carriers, hotels, and retail-related companies have slided in recent weeks. Investment analysts and economists have slashed economic growth and prospects of Asian countries, with some of them describing the SARS outbreak as biggest crisis for the Asian economy since the Asian Crisis of 1998. Morgan Stanley cuts its economic growth of Asian economies from 5.1 percent to 4.5 percent, with its Chief Economist, Stephen Roach, predicting a world recession due to the SARS fears. Stocks of technology companies and Asian high tech firms have also taken a beating. For China, the government's lack of transparency in the handling of SARS epidemic has dented investors confidence in investing in the country.

Booming Pharmaceutical Industries

However, some industries and business have benefited from the outbreak of SARS. Makers and manufacturers of surgical face masks are working their factories to meet the increased demand. So are manufacturers of hygiene products such as disinfectant aerosols. These products are flying off the shelves of supermarkets and pharmacies. Chinese medicine stores have also seen their business tripling.

This arises from the purported health benefits of some Chinese medicine in preventing the catching of SARS virus. As a result, stocks of pharmaceutical and health products companies, such as 3M, Japan Vilene and ICN Pharmaceuticals, have seen their stocks climb by as high as 18 percent.

Besides the voluntary use of face masks by people — airports, companies and even governments have started to make the wearing of face masks mandatory. Thailand has made it mandatory for that all travellers from SARS-affected countries to wear a face mask at all times while in Thailand or face a hefty fine.

While individual health insurance policies cover SARS-related treatment and hospitalisation, insurance claims filed to cover business losses related to SARS may not be applicable. "Business interruption" insurance claims may not apply according to some insurers. Policies such as quarantine imposed by the government is also not covered.

Strain on Health-Care System

In addition to the economic cost of SARS, the social cost is also being felt heavily. In Hong Kong — where the number of cases is rising rapidly and most of the SARS-affected patients being medical staff — the health care system is being stretched to its limit. Hong Kong is racing to open new isolation wards. The Health

Authority is busily converting the Prince Margaret Hospital in the densely-populated Kowloon district into a special center with isolation wards to handle up to 500 SARS cases. Contingency plans are also being drawn up to convert a second hospital into isolation wards.

However, there are no plans to fly victims out of Hong Kong yet. Nurses and health-care workers have cancelled leave and are working overtime. In addition, they are subjecting themselves to the high risk of contracting SARS. Hospitals are also discharging and transferring non-SARS patients to other hospitals for the isolation of SARS victims. Should the number of people affected by SARS increase sharply, the health-care system may collapse and be rendered unable to cope.

In Toronto, hospitals are also slapped with rising medical costs needed for the treatment of SARS patients and are looking to the Ministry of Health for funding. Elective surgery has been cancelled at all Toronto-area hospitals. The over-burdened health-care system in Toronto is also under additional strain from the quarantine of many of its health care workers and patients.

NEVER TOO OLD A REMEDY

An Exclusive Interview with Professor Leung Ping Chung

When the phone call to Professor Leung Ping-Chung's residence in Hong Kong was put through, it was close to midnight. In spite of a long day's work combating the deadly atypical pneumonia at Prince of Wales Hospital, one of the hardest hit hospitals in the Special Administrative Region of China, the microsurgery and hand surgery specialist's voice gave no trace of fatigue.

Before one could query him on his "discovery" in using serum from recovered patients to treat SARS victims, he was quick to point out that it was an old remedy that has been frequently used. What he did, he said, was merely to apply that flexibly. His calm manner belies the fact that many lives are saved as a result of this ingenuity.

The atypical pneumonia recently labelled as Severe Acute Respiratory Syndrome or SARS has taken many parts of the world by storm. Amid the constant stream of grim news, smooth recovery of patients due to Professor Leung's trial certainly stood out, bringing joy and hope to many. Such smooth recovery leads doctors to believe that some people with the respiratory disease have been able to produce antibodies, which are found in serum, to fight the illness. This is contrary to experts' earlier assumption and fear that this would not happen as the body might not easily develop antibodies.

The presence of antibodies in turn implies that those who have recovered would have developed some level of immunity against the illness in the future.

Professor Leung said that as SARS is a new disease, no one is certain of the strain of virus that causes it. Since some patients do not respond to the cocktail of anti-virals and steroids prescribed for most SARS victims, the decision was made to extract serum from recovered patients and use it on such patients. However, he stressed that only critically ill patients, such as those being put into the Intensive Care Units or those who are found to be lacking in oxygen, need to undergo such form of treatment. To date, a third of the SARS patients in Hong Kong have undergone the treatment.

Touching on the subject of a possibility that a patient's body may reject the antibodies in the recovered patient's serum, Professor Leung said: "This method is different from blood transfusion, and such a possibility is rather low."

In order to gain insights into how other territories are treating SARS, this chair professor of orthopaedics at Chinese University of Hong Kong travelled north to visit several hospitals, which have witnessed SARS cases. The personal visits have led him to conclude that while the condition in Guangzhou has not been fully arrested, it has scaled down from its peak when it saw some 1000 cases. This in turn meant that the Mainlanders would have done something right. Thus, Professor Leung suggested that Hong Kong joins hands with China to heighten prevention.

In a commentary entitled "Preventing a Pestilence" which he contributed to the press, Professor Leung pointed out that although there continues to be a geographical divide between Hong Kong and China, an increase in trans-border travels has blurred such divide. He added that in considering healthcare and preventive measures to stop a pestilence, the concept of a border "exists only in name".

As a matter of fact, Professor Leung has walked the talk. Apart from his accolades in medical research and education, he has participated in community work actively and helped set up several recuperation centres in China.

The amiable Professor became more reserved when asked to comment on the different research findings that traced the beginning of the epidemic to different viruses. It is best to wait for the announcement from the World Health Organisation, he said.

"They are too quick in commenting on the mode of viral transmission. We should not discuss this now; devising ways to stop the virus from spreading is a more critical thing to do."

He is perturbed with the Hong Kong government's delay in stepping up precautionary measures, although China's Guangdong province has witnessed atypical pneumonia as early as November 2002. He had earlier criticised the Hong Kong government for its attempt in playing down the seriousness of the illness and its inability to learn from China's experience.

He had earlier asked: "Does Hong Kong want to follow in Guangzhou's footstep? The first SARS case appeared in November 2002, but the virus continued to infect people for the next four months. As we worry about a fall in tourists' arrival, do we quickly address that or do we wait for another four months?"

While the Hong Kong government subsequently announced a series of measures to prevent the disease from spreading, including making it compulsory for people who have come in close contact with patients to go for checkups; closing kindergartens, primary and secondary schools for nine days, and putting people from the Amoy Gardens in quarantine, many Hongkongers dismissed these as exercising damage control. But Professor Leung declined comments on these measures, reiterating the need to instead devise ways to stop the virus from spreading.

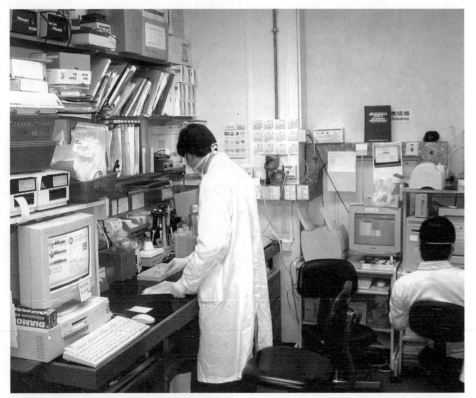

Scientists at work at the Prince of Wales Hospital.

As of April 2, the number of SARS cases in Hong Kong was more than 700, culminating in 16 deaths.

Professor Leung, who takes a keen interest in traditional Chinese medicine, said that there has not been evidence on whether Chinese medicine can be used to cure the illness, although both Chinese and Western medicine has been used concurrently in China. He is also of the view that the circulation of different concoctions of Chinese herbs in the market may not be at all bad, for the herbs are consumed for preventive purposes and "should be harmless".

It is also noteworthy that Professor Leung has remained optimistic in the fight against SARS. He observed that those who died had other illnesses and is confident that the problem can be arrested.

"It appears that the virus involved is similar to that which caused the common flu. In many instances, the disease did not develop into pneumonia. Perhaps we can call it a very bad flu."

Having to work with patients all day long to help combat the potent disease, Professor Leung is most aware of the pain and suffering that a patient undergoes. So, what precautions does he personally take to avoid being infected?

Said this highly respected medical professional: "In choosing to be a doctor, I have long had little regards for such things!"

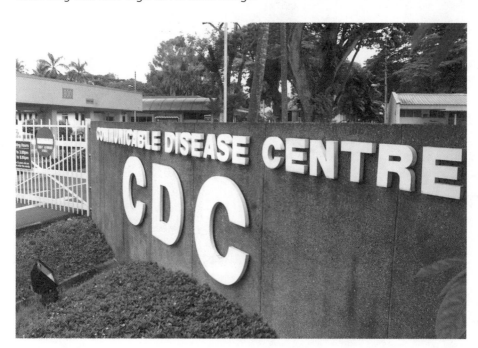

Meanwhile, Singapore announced on the April 1 that its doctors have started to use serum on a critically ill patient. Although things seem to be looking up, doctors are cautious about jumping into conclusions at an early stage. They are also exploring whether more SARS patients should undergo the treatment.

Dr Leo Yee Sin, the clinical director of Singapore's Communicable Disease Centre, told reporters that although the organisation has tried ways and means to cure the particular patient, none proved effective; it thus decided to try using serum. She added that the patient was initially 100% reliant on respiratory aids but that dependence fell to 90% after serum was used.

The patient* had received the serum from one of the recovered SARS patients. Doctors first took blood from this person, separated serum from the red blood cells before returning the latter to the person and only used 300 ml of serum.

Dr Leo disclosed that 300 ml of serum was just sufficient for a person's usage and a person can only donate his serum once in a week. Other words of caution: Not every person who has recovered could donate his serum. The donor and the recipient have to first belong to the same blood group and the former's blood has to be cleared of other viruses and found to have sufficient proteins.

In addition, said Dr Leo, not every patient can undergo such treatment, as there can be cases of rejection which may cause a patient's health to deteriorate. She added that some 90% of patients depend on their immune system to fight the virus and it is unnecessary to use serum on them. She said that as Hong Kong has experienced more SARS cases and have successfully used serum in many cases, Singapore doctors would continue to learn from them.

---

* Unfortunately, the patient passed away due to other complications.

STARRING IN SARS
Super Infectors

SARS is a lot more infectious than originally thought – such were the words from Singapore's Health Minister Lim Hng Kiang as he stepped into the room filled with reporters on March 31.

It was the same room that top health personnel of the island meets regularly to discuss health matters that affect everyone in the country. Since the middle of March, however, it has doubled up as the venue where health experts and representatives from relevant departments field questions from the press, giving them updates on developments in the severe acute respiratory syndrome or SARS.

Mr Lim maintained that SARS is spread by droplets discharged when a person sneezes or coughs and that transmission is restricted to having close contact with the infected person – defined as within a 3-feet (about 1-metre) radius or two rows in front and behind the person in an aircraft.

Singapore General Hospital virologist Ling Ai Ee explained that such droplets are heavier than the airborne ones which are so light that they "can be blown down the corridor". Examples of airborne particles are found in tuberculosis and measles, while droplets are spotted in influenza.

Still, SARS can be very infectious. Mr Lim emphasised that the disease in question is a new one and information on it is being disseminated at all times. He added that the assessment that SARS is more infectious is enhanced by the presence of what is termed "super infectors".

These are people who are "full of the virus" and are capable of infecting a large pool of people. Such characteristic has been prevalent in Hanoi and Hong Kong too, Mr Lim said. One of the first super infector beyond Singapore, for example, was the American-Chinese who had given the virus to more than 50 people and led to the closure of the Hanoi French Hospital in Vietnam, another could be the man responsible for infecting many others in the Amoy Gardens apartment building in Hong Kong, added Mr Lim.

Out of the over 90 SARS patients in Singapore, three have been identified to be super infectors. Of the first three index cases that contracted the disease from Hong Kong's Metropole Hotel, Mr Lim elaborated, only one by the name of Esther Mok is a super infector. She infected 20 people in five days, including her parents who passed away, while the two others who brought the virus back from Hong Kong have not infected anyone and have since recovered and discharged from the hospital.

The second Singapore super infector was a nurse who was infected by Esther Mok. She caught the virus when Singapore was still largely unaware of SARS and did not isolate her. The nurse subsequently passed the virus to 16 people, including Madam Painah Abdullah who died on March 30. Madam Painah was Super Infector Number Three and had infected more than 20 others.

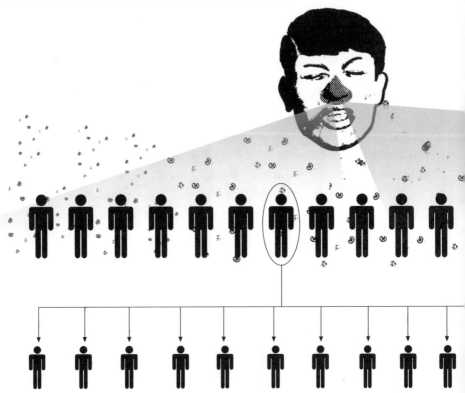

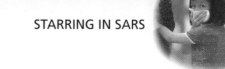

Mr Lim said that the presence of super infectors, coupled with the discovery that the coronavirus – the family of virus that SARS is believed to belong – can stay in the environment for up to three hours, implied that "the whole picture can be quite different".

"If index cases are not super infectors, the situation will not be so drastic, but Singaporeans cannot be lulled into complacency. The problem cannot be stopped next week and we will still continue to face new index cases. If any of the new index cases is a super infector, we can have a new huge cluster of infected people to start a chain of reactions," cautioned Mr Lim.

As of April 3, the number of index cases climbed to seven, most having gone to Hong Kong and China and contracted the virus there. No news on whether these are super infectors yet.

Mr Lim added that in the same way that some people are very good hosts and some are not, the former have a lot of viruses in them. If they are kept in the Intensive Care Unit, their chances of infecting people are lower than if they are moving around in the community.

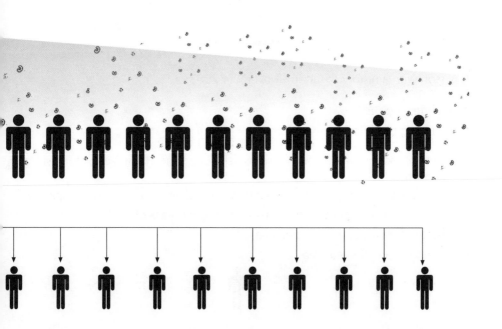

The characteristics of super infectors have, however, not been identified, although Dr Ling Ai Ee said that could be due to pre-conditions such as lung problem or that the patients are already weak in one way constitutionally, such as in the case of a diabetic.

So, Dr Ling advised that the best thing to do is to identify those who are sick very quickly. In a separate press briefing that she chaired on April 2, she disclosed that the blood of an index case in Singapore was sent to the Centres for Disease Control and Prevention (CDC) in Atlanta and it is evident that it is linked to a case in Hanoi. Besides, polymerase chain reaction (PCR), a molecular test to detect minute amounts of viral DNA or RNA, performed on a primary patient in Singapore found sequences exactly the same as that posted by CDC for a patient who died in Bangkok.

Dr Ling said that such links are important to ascertain that health authorities in different places are more or less dealing with the same thing. A link has, however, not been established with Hong Kong yet.

She added that while the jury is still out with some laboratories having found the paramyxovirus, some coronavirus and yet others discovering both viruses in SARS patients, "the consensus is leaning towards the coronavirus". Identifying the parts of the coronavirus genes that are unique is a key step in developing anti-viral and vaccines. Coming out with a diagnostic kit is equally significant.

Currently, the World Health Organisation's case definitions for SARS are as follow:

Suspect Case

A person with a history of (after 1 November 2003) :

- high fever (>38°C)
- coughing or difficulty breathing

AND one or more of the following exposures during the 10 days prior to onset of symptoms:
- close contact (having cared for, lived with, or had direct contact with respiratory secretions or body fluids of) a suspect or probable case of SARS
- history of travel, to an affected area
- residing in an affected area

Probable Case

- A suspect case with chest x-ray findings of pneumonia or Respiratory Distress Syndrome

OR

- A suspect case with an unexplained respiratory illness resulting in death, with an autopsy examination demonstrating the pathology of Respiratory Distress Syndrome without an identifiable cause.

So, what are the best precautionary measures?

Ordinary ones that protect people from the common cold virus or influenza virus should work against SARS, Dr Ling said. Wash hands a lot – "soap and water is fine" as coronavirus cannot withstand any sort of detergent – keep hands away from one's face and avoid crowded places.

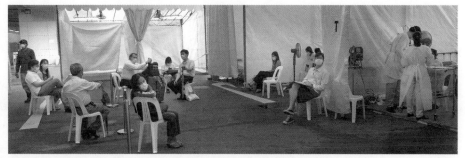

Developing diagnostic kits to ascertain that patients have SARS is pertinent.
(Source: Straits Times)

FROM THE GROUND
Real Life Accounts

Healthcare Workers Shunned by Public

Medical personnel who are risking their lives to attend to SARS patients are unexpectedly finding themselves being shunned by the general public.

A nurse who works at the Tan Tock Seng Hospital said in an interview with the media that she is disappointed with the reaction of the public. She disclosed that this is the first time in her forty years of nursing career that she has witnessed medical workers being ostracised.

She said, "When we are in our hospital uniforms, people are afraid to sit beside us in buses or the MRT." She also cited instances of commuters throwing disapproving glances or even pointing fingers at them.

It seems that it was no better even if they chose to travel by taxis. Some healthcare workers, having experienced the difficulty of stopping taxis when they are in hospital uniforms, have resorted to changing to normal clothes before they leave the hospital.

Hospital administration staff are not spared either.

An administrator, who works in the same hospital, has been asked by friends to refrain from attending a birthday party, for fear that other people might become worried or anxious. The reason given is that she is working in the hospital that is tasked to combat the deadly disease. Her friends have even requested her to conceal her identity if she insists on attending the function.

She has decided not to attend.

"When we are in our hospital uniforms, people are afraid to sit beside us in buses or the MRT."

Risking Their Lives to Save Others

At a time when everyone is living in fear of SARS, medical personnel are at the frontline battling to save lives and care for the patients who are down with the virus. Unfortunately, some of them are infected in the course of their work, although all possible precautions have been taken.

Ms. Tan, a Singaporean nurse, fell sick and was warded soon after attending to a SARS patients. Fortunately, her condition stabilised very quickly. While still recuperating from the illness, she was already rearing to re-join her colleagues in the battle against the SARS virus.

In another case, a nursing student came down with the flu-like disease in early March when the outbreak was still not very widespread. She did not seek medical attention immediately after developing a fever. For six days, her high fever came on and off. It was only until her temperature had reached 40°C that her mother sent her to the Accident and Emergency department of the Tan Tock Seng Hospital.

The doctors warded her at once. For the three days that followed, her condition worsened and she developed a very bad cough. She would cough uncontrollably even while drinking water. She was then sent to the isolation ward. In an interview with reporters later, she said, "Once the respirator is taken off, I will cough very badly." She also described herself as very tired and depressed, and felt like she was dying.

After 12 days in hospital, she recovered and was well enough to go home. Looking back, she could not understand why she had caught the disease. She believed that she was infected by one of the index cases, but she had very little contact with that patient. Her colleague, who was looking after the index patient, was not infected though.

The Tan Tock Seng Hospital, which is tasked to specifically handle SARS cases, have implemented precautionary measures very early on to prevent its medical staff from catching the virus. All personnel who come into contact with SARS patients have to wear surgical face masks, protective garb and gloves. Before they leave the

While still recuperating from the illness, she was already rearing to re-join her colleagues in the battle against the SARS virus.

wards, they have to discard the gloves and garb. They are also required to wash and disinfect their hands.

Doctors and nurses who look after non-SARS patients are required to wear surgical face masks and wash and disinfect their hands as well. Pregnant healthcare workers are not deployed to attend to SARS cases.

Amoy Gardens Residents Isolated

In the early morning of 31 March 2003, the Hong Kong Government issued an urgent "isolation order": To seal off the hundreds of residents in Amoy Garden Block E.

6 a.m.: Many residents of Amoy Garden Block E were still sound asleep, oblivious to the fact that their block was going to be isolated. More than ten police cars quietly advanced towards the block, and more than a hundred policemen surrounded it, prohibiting anyone form entering or exiting the building. The policemen all donned face masks and gloves, as if facing an imminent biological war. About 200 staff from Hong Kong Department of Health and other government agencies — all garbed in protective white gowns, caps, face masks and gloves — entered the building to issue an isolation order to every family unit. The residents realised that they would be locked up at home for 10 days, and their daily meals would be delivered by the government. They would temporarily lose their freedom and would be isolated from society and the outside world.

Of the 700 residents in 264 units of the building, only 108 family units comprising 241 residents were isolated. By evening time, the government staff were able to track only half the number of residents. In other words, hundreds of people with the potential to infect others were still out on the streets.

As of 31 March 2003, of the 610 people infected with SARS in Hong Kong, 185 of the confirmed cases and 8 of the suspected cases were from Amoy Gardens, that is, 1 out of 3 people infected in Hong Kong came from Amoy Gardens. Why was the virus able to spread so quickly in Amoy Gardens?

As residents from neighbouring blocked peered out of their windows to watch, health officials, clad in protective garbs, worked tirelessly to find out how the infection had spread so rapidly to so many residents. As the virus could be spread through human excreta, the staff did not rule out the possibility that the sewage system could be a culprit. All vertically-linked common facilities at the apartment block

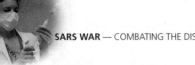

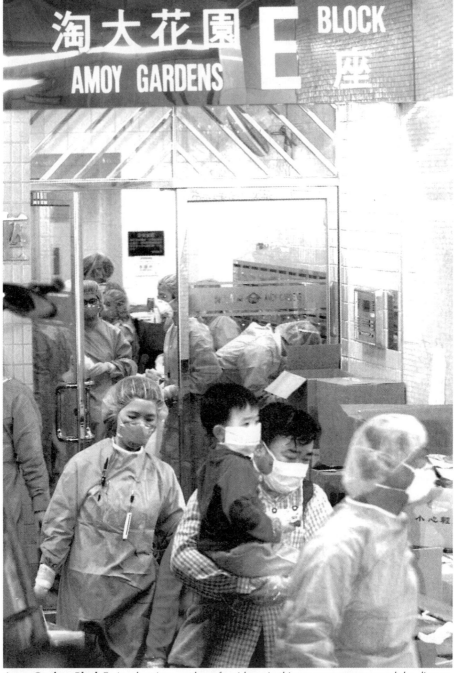

Amoy Gardens Block E *An alarming number of residents in this apartment contracted the disease, prompting the authorities to quarantine the entire building.*
(Source: Mingpao, Hong Kong)

Possible source of infection: The sewage system?

also came under scrutiny.

Also included in their investigation was the drainage system and air ventilation system which were found to be interconnected. The purpose of the interconnection was to facilitate air flow in the sewage system to ensure proper drainage. However, should the drainage system be badly maintained, the accumulated debris would clog up the system, rendering it incapable of flushing properly and resulting in the diffusion of foul air through the air ventilation system into the housing units of Block E. The consequence would be the spread of the SARS virus to the adjacent units as well as the interconnecting units.

In addition, experts have pointed out that the letter-boxes serving units 7 and 8 of the Block E are interconnected and could be another possible route for transmission of the virus.

As scientists are still unsure of the exact mode of transmission of the SARS virus, the Hong Kong government fears that an outbreak as severe as the one in Amoy Gardens might occur again anytime, transforming a whole block or even an entire neighbourhood into a deadly epicentre of infection.

Quarantined!

Due to the highly contagious nature of SARS, many governments have to resort to quarantine as a means of containing the disease. The reactions of those who had to be confined to their homes have been mixed: while some lamented at the sudden loss of personal freedom, others took the opportunity to rest and spend time with their families.

The Hong Kong authorities decided to quarantine the residents of Block E of the Amoy Gardens apartment when it was found that more than 250 cases of infection were detected among them.

Some residents have complained that being confined to their homes was worse than being in jail, as even prisoners are allocated time for outdoor activities. Another complaint was that the daily rations provided by the government were unpalatable. One resident who declined to be named was particularly annoyed by the fact that he was "not even given any butter" to go with the bread for breakfast.

As the quarantine was imposed suddenly, some families became separated as some residents were not in the apartment compounds when the police sealed off the place. Some of them had had to plead with the authorities to be allowed to return to their homes so that they could help take care of their children or the elderly in their families.

In Singapore, the government invoked the Infectious Disease Act, and

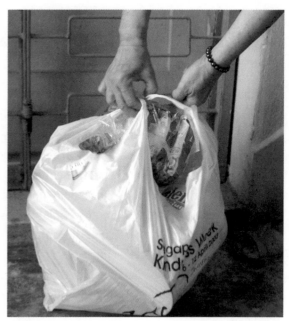

Grocery Shopping *Many quarantined people have to resort to asking friends and relatives to do grocery shopping for them. To ensure minimal contact, grocery bags are left at the door.*

quarantined all the people who came into close contact with infected cases, for 10 days.

Many families were caught unprepared, and had to resort to asking family members or friends to supply them with daily groceries and necessities. However, the advent of the Internet has made online shopping possible, so grocery shopping during the quarantine period did not really pose a problem.

Some people adopted a positive attitude towards the quarantine. One such person was Mr. Wong. In a telephone interview with a radio station, he said that the members in his family were usually busy with their own work, and had little time for interaction. Ironically, the quarantine period provided his family with a valuable opportunity to take a break and spend some quality time with one another. He jovially said, "… at least this is a blessing in disguise!"

Ironically, the quarantine period provided his family with a valuable opportunity to take a break and spend some quality time with one another.

However, people from the lower income group, especially those who received daily wages, were frustrated that they could not report for work. A blue-collar worker lamented, "I'm the sole bread winner in the family but now I'm stuck at home. My kids need me to go out and work to bring home the dough!"

"I'm the sole bread winner in the family but now I'm stuck at home. My kids need me to go out and work to bring home the dough!"

FREQUENTLY ASKED QUESTIONS

1. **What is Severe Acute Respiratory Syndrome (atypical pneumonia)?**

SARS is a newly emerging infections respiratory illness (atypical pneumonia) of unknown cause that has been recently reported globally. The illness begins generally with a rapid rise of fever (above 38 degrees Celsius) and cough. It is also characterised by muscle ache, chills, soar throat, diarrhoea and headache.

Other less common symptoms include diarrhoea and skin rashes. In small number of cases the disease may be followed by difficulty in breathing and may progress to a severe form of pneumonia and even death. The illness is associated with history of travel to the affected areas or close contact with persons who had diagnosed with SARS.

2. **What causes severe acute respiratory syndrome?**

Scientists at the CDC in Atlanta and several other places have regarded coronavirus as the leading hypothesis for the etiology of SARS. However, it is still premature at this stage to confirm if this is true.

Coronavirus — one of the strains is the cause of common flu — can survive in the environment for up to three hours. Coronaviruses infect humans and many animal species including poultry, turkeys, cows, rabbits, dogs, rats, mice and pigs. Several human coronavirus strains cause about 10-20% of all common colds. They are enveloped viruses which are fragile, and easily killed by soaps and detergents.

3. **Is it contagious, and how is it spread?**

Yes, it is contagious. From SARS cases seen so far, it spreads through close contact (history of having cared from, having lived with, having face to face contact with or having had contact with respiratory secretions of a probable case).

4.   **How soon will someone become ill after getting infected?**

Typically it will take 2-7 days; however it may take as long as 10-14 days. The illness begins generally with a fever over 38 degrees Celsius followed by a dry cough 2 days later. (see above for signs and symptoms)

5.   **Is the disease fatal?**

In most cases no. With early detection and treatment there is a high chance of recovery. Severe cases are usually seen in patients with pre-existing health problems or who seek treatment at a late stage.

6.   **Who are at risk?**

Persons who have recently visited the affected areas or have been in close contact with cases of SARS.

7.   **How is SARS diagnosed?**

A diagnosis is based on clinical symptoms, history of recent travel to high risk areas or history of close contact with persons with SARS and chest x-ray.

8.   **Can it be treated?**

At the moment, there is no specific treatment. If you have recently returned from affected areas and have flu-like symptoms (see above for signs and symptoms), you should seek medical treatment as early as possible.

However, experience shows that some patients may react favourably to ribavirin (a broad spectrum antiviral drug) and steroid treatment. Other treatment methods are also being developed and tested.

9.   **Is there a vaccination for SARS?**

There is no vaccine currently available for the prevention of SARS.

10.   **Which are the high risk areas?**

According to WHO, local disease transmission is reported in the following countries: Canada - Toronto; Singapore; China - Guandong Province, Hong

Kong, Shanxi; Taiwan; and Vietnam - Hanoi, as of 5th April 2003.
Note: The countries included in the above table will change according to the World Health Organisation daily update.

As a precautionary measure, travel to those affected areas should be avoided unless absolutely necessary. For those who are unable to delay their travel to these places, they are advised to avoid crowded places, observe strict personal hygiene particularly hand washing and to build up the body's resistance by ensuring that you get adequate rest, proper diet and exercise.

11. What should you do if you have recently travelled to an affected area where cases of SARS have been reported?

You should monitor your own health whilst in the affected area and for the next 14 days following your return. If you become ill with a fever that is accompanied by a cough or difficulty in breathing you should go to the Accident and Emergency Department of the nearest hospital for medical treatment. Tell the doctor about your recent travel to SARS affected areas and whether you were in contact with someone who had symptoms.

12. What is the difference between classical/typical pneumonia and atypical pneumonia?

Classical/typical pneumonia is mainly caused by bacteria such as streptococcus. Atypical pneumonia is mainly caused by viruses such as influenza and adenovirus, bacteria such as chlamydia and mycoplasma, and other unknown agents.

13. What is the difference between influenza and atypical pneumonia?

Influenza symptoms such as fever, cough and headache usually subside within a few days without any serious complications or signs of pneumonia.

14. How is severe acute respiratory syndrome transmitted?

Transmission is by respiratory droplets and direct contact with a patient's secretions.

15.   Is there any evidence to suggest air-borne transmission?

Based on available information, and the results of scientific analysis, transmission is most consistent with droplets and direct contact with a patient's secretions.

16.   Is it safe to use public swimming pools?

There is no evidence of transmission through swimming. As a precautionary measure, you could avoid public pools. In any case, people feeling unwell should not go swimming.

17.   Can the disease be contracted by handling money?

There is no evidence of transmission through handling money. However, people should pay careful attention to their personal hygiene and wash hands frequently.

18.   What steps can be taken to help prevent contracting the disease?

Maintain good personal hygiene: cover your nose and mouth with a tissue when sneezing or coughing, and wash hands immediately afterwards with liquid soap.
Use a disposable towel or a hand dryer to dry hands.
   Develop a healthy lifestyle - proper diet, regular exercise, adequate rest and do not smoke.
 Ensure good ventilation at home and in the office.
   People with respiratory tract infections, or those caring for them, should wear a face mask.
Consult your doctor promptly if you develop symptoms of a respiratory infection.

19.   How can I avoid contracting the disease in an office setting?

If feeling unwell, employees should seek early medical advice and not go to work. All staff should maintain good personal hygiene and a healthy lifestyle. The office should be well ventilated, and windows opened from time to time. Air conditioners should be well maintained and cleaned regularly. Office furniture and equipment should be kept clean.

20. How can I prevent contracting the disease in a lift?

Maintain good personal hygiene. Wash hands frequently. Cover your nose and mouth with a tissue when sneezing or coughing. Wear a face mask if you have symptoms of a respiratory tract infection. Building management should ensure lifts and public access areas are kept clean - lift control panels and door handles should be thoroughly and frequently cleaned with disinfectant or a diluted bleach.

21. Should I take any precautions when visiting a health care facility?

Advice has been issued to all doctors on the prevention of spreading the disease in health care settings. People seeking medical consultation should maintain good personal hygiene. Wash hands frequently. Wear a face mask.

22. What precautions should be adopted if a family member or friend has contracted the disease?

People should avoid visiting patients with atypical pneumonia. People who have close contact with patients suffering from the disease should:
- Observe quarantine regulations. You will be required to stop work, stay at home and report daily to surveillance centres for 10 days.
- If you must leave your home, wear a face mask and observe good personal hygiene.
- If you think you may have had contact with an infected person, wear a face mask for at least 10 days and seek medical advice.
- At home, clean toys and furniture properly (using a solution of 1 part bleach 49 parts water).
- Pay special attention to your health and hygiene. Wash hands frequently.
- Seek early medical advice if feeling unwell.

23. Should clothes be washed after visiting hospitals?

Yes. Wash them immediately you get home.

24. What is the advice about sharing food at home or in restaurants?

Do not share eating utensils. Adopt the good practice of using serving spoons and chopsticks.

25.   Can the disease be prevented by wearing a face mask?

Yes, a face mask can help prevent the transmission of the disease. Make sure hands are washed before putting on a mask.

26.   Who should wear a face mask?

The following people should wear a face mask:
- People with respiratory infection symptoms
- People who care for patients with respiratory infection symptoms
- People who have been in close contact with confirmed cases of atypical pneumonia should wear a face mask for at least 10 days from the last contact
- Health care workers

27.   What type of face mask should be used?

An ordinary surgical face mask is effective in preventing the spread of droplet infections.

28.   Is the N95 face mask the only effective model to prevent atypical pneumonia?

Surgical face masks and the N95 face mask are both effective in preventing the spread of droplet infections.

29.   How often should a face mask be replaced?

In general, a surgical face mask needs to be changed daily. However, replace the face mask immediately if it becomes worn or damaged.

30.   I have booked a tour to the affected countries. Should I continue with my plans?

As a precautionary measure, the advice is for you to avoid travel to Hong Kong, Guangdong Province, Taiwan, Singapore, Hanoi and Toronto (Canada) for the time being, unless absolutely necessary. For those who are unable to delay their travel to these places, you are advised to avoid crowded places and to build up your body's resistance by ensuring that you get adequate rest, proper diet and exercise.

31. **Are there any preventive injections that I could have or medications that I can take along with me before I continue with my travel plans to the affected countries?**

As the cause of the infections is not yet known, there are no specific measures that can be taken. If you are unable to delay your travel plans, you are advised to avoid crowded places and to build up your body's resistance by ensuring that you get adequate rest, proper diet and exercise.

Acknowledgement

Hong Kong Department of Health Website
Singapore Ministry of Health Website

CONTACT DETAILS

HONG KONG

Department of Health
http://www.info.gov.hk/dh/apcontent.htm

Central Health Education Unit
24-hour Health Education Hotline: 2833 0111

Education and Manpower Bureau Hotline : 2892 2352

Social Welfare Department Hotline : 2343 2255

Notification of Infections

Regional Office	Telephone Number
Hong Kong	2961 8729
Kowloon	2199 9149
New Territories East	2158 5107
New Territories West	2615 8571

Hospitals & Institutions Hotlines

Hospital Name	Phone Number
Alice Ho Miu Ling Nethersole Hospital	2689 2000
Bradbury Hospice	2636 0163
Caritas Medical Centre	3408 7911
Castle Peak Hospital	2456 7111
Cheshire Home, Chung Hom Kok	2813 9823
Cheshire Home, Shatin	2636 7288
Duchess of Kent Children's Hospital at Sandy Bay	2817 7111
Grantham Hospital	2518 2111
HK Red Cross Blood Transfusion Service	2710 1333
Haven of Hope Hospital	2703 8000
Hong Kong Buddhist Hospital	2339 6111
Hong Kong Eye Hospital	2762 3007
Kowloon Hospital	3129 7111
Kwai Chung Hospital	2959 8111
Kwong Wah Hospital	2332 2311
MacLehose Medical Rehabilitation Centre	2817 0018
Nam Long Hospital	2903 0000
North District Hospital	2683 8888
Our Lady of Maryknoll Hospital	2320 2121
Pamela Youde Nethersole Eastern Hospital	2595 6111
Pok Oi Hospital	2478 2556
Prince of Wales Hospital	2632 2211
Princess Margaret Hospital	2990 1111
Queen Elizabeth Hospital	2958 8888
Queen Mary Hospital	2855 3838
Rehabaid Centre	2364 2345
Ruttonjee Hospital	2291 2000
Shatin Hospital	2636 7500
Siu Lam Hospital	3127 0202
St. John Hospital	2981 9441
TWGHs Wong Tai Sin Hospital	2320 0377

Tai Po Hospital	2607 6111
Tang Shiu Kin Hospital	2291 2000
Tsan Yuk Hospital	2589 2100
Tseung Kwan O Hospital	2208 0111
Tuen Mun Hospital	2468 5111
Tung Wah Eastern Hospital	2162 6888
Tung Wah Group of Hospital	
- Fung Yiu King Hospital	2855 6111
Tung Wah Hospital	2589 8111
United Christian Hospital	2379 4000
Wong Chuk Hang Hospital	2873 7222
Yan Chai Hospital	2417 8383

Private Hospitals Hotlines

Region	Hospital (24-hr service)	Telephone No.
Hong Kong Island	Canossa Hospital (Caritas)	2522 2181
	Hong Kong Adventist Hospital	2574 6211
	Hong Kong Central Hospital	2522 3141
	HK Sanatorium & Hospital Limited	2572 0211
	Matilda & War Memorial Hospital	2849 0111
	St. Paul's Hospital	2890 6008
Kowloon	Evangel Hospital	2711 5221
	Hong Kong Baptist Hospital	2339 8888
	Precious Blood Hospital (Caritas)	2386 4281
	St. Teresa' Hospital	2200 3434
New Territories	Shatin International Medical Centre	
	Union Hospital	2608 3388
	Tsuen Wan Adventist Hospital	2276 7676

CHINA

Ministry of Health of China
http://www.moh.gov.cn
Tel: 8610-68792114
Email: manage@chsi.moh.gov.cn

SINGAPORE

Ministry of Health
http://app.moh.gov.sg

General info on SARS: 1-800-2254122
(8.00am – 11.00pm daily)

Enquiries on closure of schools, MOE hotline: 6872-2220

Enquiries on closure of childcare and student care centres, MCDS hotline: 1800-2580677

Ambulance deployment for suspected SARS cases, please call: 91788477 / 91788478
Email: MOH_info@moh.gov.sg

Hospitals

* Changi General Hospital

  http://www.cgh.com.sg

  General Enquiry: 67888833
  Accident & Emergency (24 hours): 68501680

* Tan Tock Seng Hospital
  http://www.ttsh.com.sg
  Main Line: 62566011
  General Enquiries/ Patient Relations Services (toll-free): 1800-2529919

Emergency (A & E) Department: 63578866
Communicable Disease Centre: 63577900

- Singapore General Hospital
http://www.sgh.com.sg
General Enquiries (24 hours): 62223322
Patient Enquiries: 63266933
Accident & Emergency (24 hours): 63214311
Urgent Matters (after office hours): 62223322

HANOI, VIETNAM

Ministry of Health
138A Giang Vo Str., Hanoi
Health Department: 844-82-62-415

TAIWAN

Center for Disease Control Taiwan, R.O.C.
http://www.cdc.gov.tw/en/
No.6, Linshen S. Rd., Taipei, Taiwan 100, R.O.C.
886-2-2395-9825

CANADA

Health Canada
http://www.hc-sc.gc.ca/english/protection/warnings/2003/2003_11.htm

Public: 1-800-454-8302
Airport passengers seeking further information: 1-800-454-8302

Ontario Ministry of Health and Long-Term Care
http://www.health.gov.on.ca
For general information about SARS, call INFOline at: 1-888-668-4636
(TTY 1-866-797-0007).
If you have symptoms of SARS, call Telehealth Ontario at: 1-866-797-0000
(TTY 1-800-387-5559).

USA

Centers for Disease Control and Prevention
http://www.cdc.gov/ncidod/sars/

Public: English 888-246-2675
            Español 888-246-2857
            TTY 866-874-2646
Clinician: English 877-554-4625

WORLD HEALTH ORGANISATION

http://www.who.int/crs/sars/en/